Wisdom From Five Cancer Travelers: Lessons Learned

Wisdom From Five Cancer Travelers: Lessons Learned
ISBN 978-1-7373694-5-5   Hardbound
ISBN 978-1-7373694-6-2   Softbound
ISBN 978-1-7373694-7-9   E-Book
Copyright © 2021. Richard Farmer
All rights reserved.

No parts of this publication may be reproduced, stored in a retrieval system, or transmitted in any form or by any means, electronic, mechanical, photocopying, recording, or otherwise, without the prior written permission of the copyright owner.

This book is sold subject to the condition that it shall not, by way of trade or otherwise, be lent, resold, hired out, or otherwise circulated without the publisher's prior consent in any form of binding or cover other than that in which it is published and without a similar condition including this condition being imposed on the subsequent purchaser. Under no circumstances may any part of this book be photocopied for resale.

Cover by Alex Cotton *(Unrelenting Media)*
Editing & Formatting by Joniece Jackson

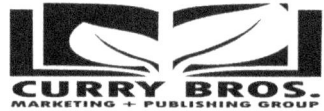

Table of Contents

Preface..1

Chapter One. Being A Cancer Patient...7

Chapter Two. Obtaining Support..41

Chapter Three. Hope..65

Chapter Four. Saying Goodbye..87

Chapter Five. A Meaningful Life...117

Epilogue. Lessons Learned...147

Preface

This book is the result of the experiences of five individuals as they have coped with a cancer diagnosis. Reflections by each author's personal experience with cancer are presented, in their own words, based on five common themes in the format of essays, vignettes, and short stories designed to illustrate the theme. Each author's experience is as unique, distinct, and honest as the writers themselves.

The themes were developed by the senior author, Richard E. Farmer, as a result of his experience in coping with his cancer diagnosis and the effect cancer had upon his life. He was diagnosed with Multiple Myeloma cancer in the fall of 2014. While there is at present no known cure for this cancer, Richard is in a close state of remission due to a stem cell transplant and ongoing successful treatment with chemotherapy.

The five themes presented are: Being a Cancer Patient, Obtaining Support, Hope, Saying Goodbye, and Living a Meaningful Life. In the Epilogue, subtitled Lessons Learned, each author will briefly synthesize their most important lessons learned.

Being a Cancer Patient

In this chapter, each author describes their cancer journey starting at the pre-diagnosis stage, for some, and ending with their conclusion of treatment, chemotherapy, ongoing treatment, or enhanced surveillance. Such descriptions, for example, include intimate feelings and attitudes associated with this new status of life.

Obtaining Support

Reflections in this section include views, attitudes, and needs for support. The authors share what support means to them and how it feels when addressing how we can call on others to help us cope with our cancer. Questions pondered include can one identify support when experienced or reaching out or not to caregivers, co-workers, fellow patients, and providers to help us better develop an understanding of our new status as a cancer patient from a healthful point-of-view. Does the meaning of support change over time and how? A cancer patient who has lived with incurable cancer for six years may likely experience a change in how support is viewed or has changed throughout their course of treatments, setbacks, disease progression, decline, and recovery from acute medical-cancer events. The concept of support also raises the question of how we can reciprocate to the other members of our support group.

Hope

Hope is a critical attitude for the maintenance of positive mental health in all people and is especially critically important for a cancer patient. Possessing hope gives us the ability to purposely direct our lives in a positive direction. And hope helps us to produce a balance between living in the present and some living directed toward the future. Reflections on hope include, for example, an individual's understanding of hope and what is hoped for. Goals of hope may change over time with disease management and disease progression. Thoughts on the cancer patient nurturing hope within themselves or from others are explored.

Saying Goodbye

For most of us, our inner circle of "loved ones" could include spouses, life partners, children and grandchildren, parents and siblings, and close friends. It is with these individuals that we must face one of the most emotionally difficult tasks with saying goodbye. Saying goodbye is not necessarily restricted to the death bed with few moments to spare. For example, while medications can stop being effective, an infection can become critical. Or, if the average lifespan for a given diagnosis is three to five years, the cancer patient in year one, five years might be all one hears and sounds "pretty good". At year seven for that same patient, the same words can ring like a death knoll.

Another example of reflections by the cancer patient include, what are the words that we use to communicate that we may sooner or later die? Meaning, at the age of 58 with the prognosis for a five-year life span might imply that one may not see an infant grandchild graduate from high school, or a beloved niece get married, or a dear friend realize her dream of becoming an accomplished musician. The challenge of saying goodbye can evoke powerful reactions and responses for both the cancer patient and the recipient of the message. Emotional preparation for the cancer patients and their "inner circles" can be essential for such difficult conversations.

Living a Meaningful Life

Living a meaningful life is important for all of us and is especially important for cancer patients. As all cancer patients know, the disease can quickly destroy meaning in one's life as we attempt to cope with an all-encompassing disease. Understanding this process is vitally important for successful treatment of the disease. We need to come to terms with the fact that cancer has changed much about who we are; it robs the prior meaning we had about who and what we are, at least to some measure. Bearing this in mind, we have the knowledge and ability to reach within ourselves and choose to recreate who and what we once were to what we now want to be. Recognizing that meaningfulness is the cornerstone upon which we rebuild our lives post-diagnosis is the very first step in this process.

Epilogue - Lessons Learned

The Epilogue will provide a brief review of what each author has chosen as the most significant Lessons Learned as travelers on their reluctant cancer journey.

Meet the Authors

In addition to Richard E. Farmer, the four other authors include: David W. Persky, Bonnie Cashin Farmer, Cherie L. Genua and Burt Harres. A brief summary of their professional experiences follows.

Richard E. Farmer is the former President of the Maine College of Health Professions having retired due to his health status with Multiple Myeloma Cancer. Dr. Farmer earned an undergraduate degree from Saint Anselm College, a graduate degree from the University of New Haven, and a Doctor of Education degree from Boston University. He is a psychologist, faculty member, and academic administrator. His psychological practice has focused on stress management issues for police, first responders, and government employees. His former presidencies were at Sanford-Brown College and McIntosh College. He held senior administrative positions at Ohio Dominican University, Saint Leo University, and Providence College. He also held tenured full professorships at the University of New Haven,

Sacred Heart University, and Cape Cod Community College. Dr. Farmer is the author of three books, two book chapters, ten refereed journal articles, numerous newspaper articles and professional monographs, and a multitude of research papers presented at professional societies.

David W. Persky is a former professor of Criminal Justice at Saint Leo University. He holds an undergraduate degree from Southern Methodist University, a master's degree in Personnel Counseling from Miami University, a Ph.D. in Higher Education Administration from Florida State University, and a J.D. from Stetson University College of Law. Dr. Persky held a variety of administrative and academic positions at the University of South Florida, Florida State University and Saint Leo University. Just prior to his retirement from Saint Leo, he was diagnosed with prostate cancer. He successfully completed radiation therapy and is currently in remission.

Dr. Persky has been highly active in a variety of community service and academic honors organizations. He is a member of Civitan International and has served as club president and district governor for the organization. He has been a volunteer for Florida Special Olympics for over 40 years and served as Chair of the Education, Employment and Economic Development Committee of the Greater Tampa Chamber of Commerce. Dr. Persky served on the national executive committee of Kappa Sigma Fraternity and was elected to post of International President of Kappa Sigma in 1999. He has also been highly active in several academic honor societies: Alpha Phi Sigma Criminal Justice Honor Society, Omicron Delta Kappa National Leadership Honor Society, Blue Key and Order of Omega. He has been listed in Who's Who in the South and Southwest and in Who's Who Among American College and University Students. Lastly, Dr. Persky has been recognized for the creation and development of "My Brother's Keeper" student alcohol abuse prevention program for college Greek organizations.

Bonnie Cashin Farmer is a former tenured Associate Professor of Nursing with an emphasis in Gerontological Nursing and Leadership at the University of Southern Maine. Prior to this, she was a tenured nursing faculty member at Southern Connecticut State University. She possesses undergraduate degrees in nursing from Northeastern University and Saint Anselm College, a Master of Public Administration and Health Care Management from the University of New Haven and a Ph.D. in Nursing from the University of Rhode Island. In addition, she holds a Certificate in Geriatric Education from the University of Connecticut and an Executive Certificate in Health Policy and Management from the Harvard University School of Public Health. She retired in spring 2014 from teaching to pursue an independent project with colleagues that would advance gerontological nursing knowledge of the older adult within nursing education and ultimately clinical practice. In late fall of 2014 she became, and remains, a full-time caregiver to her spouse who was diagnosed with Multiple Myeloma cancer. In early 2015 she was diagnosed with invasive ductal breast cancer and was successfully treated with surgery, radiation, and chemotherapy. Her perspectives written in these pages come from three different viewpoints: Her own breast cancer diagnosis and successful treatment, her caregiving to her spouse, and her academic and experiential background as a nurse.

Cherie LaFlamme Genua holds a Bachelor of Arts degree in English from Southern Connecticut State University in New Haven and an MBA from the University of Massachusetts Amherst. She was diagnosed with ER+PR+HER2 + Stage 2 breast cancer (invasive ductal carcinoma) at the age of 34 and was labeled "no evidence of disease" in June of 2019.

Cherie is a passionate, committed, and devoted writer. In addition to her work on this writing project, she is in the process of completing her first fiction novel. She is an ESL literacy volunteer and enjoys hiking, traveling, and interior design. She has worked in the software development space for many years and is the Director of Product for a software company in Connecticut.

Burt Harres has had a number of faculty and university positions within the system of colleges and universities within the state of Florida. As an administrator, he served as the Chief Academic Officer for a multi-campus community college, and as Provost and Dean, Director of Financial Aid, Director of Special Services and Assistant to the President. Eventually, he earned a Bachelor of Science in Education degree from Southeast Missouri State University, a Master of Science in Education degree from Indiana University, and a Doctor of Philosophy (Ph.D.) in Higher Education Administration from the University of Florida.

Dr. Harres is a widely respected faculty member and administrator and has extensive teaching experience in Humanities, Art, Health Education and Fundamentals of Speech. He has been highly active in professional development activities within the Florida system as well as participation in a variety of civic organizations. His diagnosis and treatment of prostate cancer are detailed in his reflections.

CHAPTER ONE:

BEING A CANCER PATIENT

REFLECTIONS ON BEING A CANCER PATIENT

By
Richard E. Farmer

He then said the reason for his call was that he had some difficult news to tell me about the biopsy results from the operation a few days earlier. He said that the lab results from the initial biopsy suggested that I had cancer which turned out to be a relatively rare blood cancer called Multiple Myeloma. At that time in 2014, I would learn that Multiple Myeloma was an incurable cancer with an average lifespan of about 5 years.

This is an analysis of my journey with cancer which began in November of 2014 with my formal diagnosis of Multiple Myeloma Cancer. It actually began in the late summer and early fall of 2014 with my persistent complaining about a sore back. At the time I was a healthy 63-year-old man, husband, father, grandfather, university professor and psychologist who was currently serving as the President of the Maine College of Health Professions. Successful laminectomy surgery provided little to no relief for the ever-increasing back pain. Referral to another orthopedic surgeon resulted in an urgent kyphoplasty operation in an attempt to stop the cascade of vertebral compression fractures as apparent in the x-rays that were taken. A biopsy was also obtained by the surgeon.

Toward the end of my third postoperative day, I received an unexpected telephone call at home from my primary care physician who asked to speak with my spouse and me at the same time. As I put the phone on speaker, my wife gave me a terrifying look, the kind of which only a medical professional would give. She is a nurse and knew right away that something was terribly wrong. I got deep down inside scared. To say that the news of the diagnosis by our primary care physician was shocking is an understatement.

After we hung up the phone, we sat in our living room holding each other and cried uncontrollably. What the hell is multiple myeloma? I screamed, I cried….it was not fair. I was in good shape: I exercised regularly, ate properly, and took good care of myself – damn it! This is not supposed to happen! As I continued to rage, my beloved spouse, Bonnie, took my hand and cradled me as I cried my heart out! She petted my hair as if I were a baby and told me that we would get through it and get through it together.

She reminded me that we were married for 41 years and that we had faced our own sets of issues and crises as most married couples do. We had managed the usual, and the unusual, during our years together and that we will find the strength and courage to deal with this. "Yes, this is bad and devastating" she said, "but we are a strong couple, and we will get through this. I will be strong for you; you can lean on me."

Later that evening, it was her turn to let her emotions out. She began wailing. I held her, rocked her, and told her that I loved her very much and that whatever was in store for us, we would get through it. Finally, it was lights out and we both managed to fall asleep albeit a restless one. The next morning over coffee we both went to our iPads to learn about Multiple Myeloma and were shocked to read about this rather rare form of blood cancer.

We discovered that Multiple Myeloma resides in the red blood cells and which for a variety of reasons goes on an "attack" consuming other cells usually found in bone marrow. We looked at each other and with tears streaming down my face, I blurted out, "what in God's name are we going to say to the children and grandchildren, how are we going to tell them?" Knowing that we are a remarkably close family, Bonnie came over to me and put her arms around me and offered comforting words about coping, being strong, praying to God for help, guidance, and support. I took a deep breath, gave her a good morning kiss, and finished my coffee. Over time, we worked out a plan to talk with our children, grandchildren, and eventually my brothers and sisters. Little did we know that much, much more was yet to come.

Our primary care doctor referred us to several oncologists of considerable merit and reputation in the local and regional oncology community. Visits to each oncologist confirmed the diagnosis and we began the journey of chemotherapy and pain management. And, because my spine was crumbling and a further bone marrow biopsy took place, an aggressive regimen of chemotherapy coupled with pain control was initiated.

Our primary care doctor referred us to Helen F. Ryan, MD, the noted hematologic oncologist at the New England Cancer Specialist in Portland, Maine for an appointment. At the same time that this appointment was being established, we were able to secure a second opinion from an oncologist of significant scientific repute with Jacob P. Laubach, MD, MPP the Clinical Director of the Jerome Lipper Multiple Myeloma Center at the Dana Farber Cancer Institute in Boston.

Through all those tumultuous initial days of tests, assessments, and treatments, my back pain continued to worsen much of the time with a pain level of 10 within the classic 1–10-point scale. Pain medication helped only for a short while. Stronger pain meds were continually ordered without much improvement. Bonnie told the doctors that the pain was killing me, and it was. A pain pump was installed, and it finally controlled the pain. I remained in a significantly compromised and diminished state for many months. I would later learn that my spine had lost 50% of its vertebral height resulting in 5 inches of lost height and weight loss of approximately 50 lbs. within this short period of time.

Ironically, within two months of my diagnosis and during a routine physical and mammogram, Bonnie was diagnosed with breast cancer that required surgery, radiation, and long-term medication. And I should point out that during that same month of January 2015, I was hospitalized three times for extended periods of time for pain management and pneumonia. This left me with little or no appreciation for the heartbreaking trauma she was experiencing. While we kissed and I held her, the full comprehension of what she was experiencing was beyond my ability to comfort her and provide "care" that would have readily happened under normal circumstances. How Bonnie managed to support me realizing that I stood a good chance of dying and leaving her as a widow, I will never know. But that is the type of person that she is. She is a pillar of strength to me and ultimately to the children and family members, always providing the needed support when someone was in crisis over my disease. I am confident that she brought these same qualities to her patients, families, and nursing students. Bonnie is a unique, strong, and loving spouse who was committed to helping me manage the cancer. Her lifelong experience as a registered nurse, with a PhD in nursing, and now retired Professor of Nursing at the University of Southern Maine continues to positively influence my care and quality of life. She was determined that this bad, catastrophic, and potentially fatal news was not going to destroy us.

So here we are as a family, both husband and spouse, with cancer. The husband has been largely ineffective in providing any real support to his spouse. With vigilant screenings for breast cancer, Bonnie's prognosis is optimistic. However, knowing deep down inside that she has, or has had, breast cancer has created an aspect of her self-concept that now includes the concept that, like millions of other women, she too has had cancer. This knowledge, while clearly present, is now a permanent aspect of her self-concept and personality. And as her husband, and a psychologist to boot, I am too clearly knowledgeable that there is little I can do to help her alleviate any negative feelings that are associated with it. Although she has often expressed that she doesn't feel like a breast cancer survivor, I know different.

Now after 48 years of marriage, we are a caring, loving and committed couple. We live by a daily code of faith in God, and belief that a positive attitude will help us to survive and live a positive life for however long we have. We remain committed to one another, we believe in one another, and we deeply love one another. And in the end, we know with certainty that we will be together for as long as we can and forever afterwards.

For me as both a husband and a man, Bonnie's cancer has deeply challenged every aspect of my perceived role as provider, protector, and defender. She is my wife, and I promised on our marriage vows that I would love and honor her and take care of her as we grew together. And largely as our lives progressed, I was able to put real meaning and action behind those words of love, honor, and caring for her needs, as well as the needs of our children. Deep down inside of my psyche, Multiple Myeloma has basically changed some or much of this for me. Coming to terms with the many physical and psychological effects of this disease has caused me to reassess and REAFFIRM many, if not most, of my belief systems as a man, husband, and father.

As we reflect on our journey as a married couple with cancer, we have chosen to live a positive life and to make a deliberate decision to remain positive in the presence of catastrophic disease. We pray daily asking God to give us the strength to choose being positive. And while bad things happen to people, my spouse reminds me daily of the power of positive thinking which provides the basis for living a meaningful life of love, gratitude, and blessings.

THE PATIENT

By
David W. Persky

In the fall of 2019, I hit a milestone in my career at Saint Leo University based in Florida, just north of Tampa. I passed the 20-year mark as a member of the Saint Leo community. I loved my work, but I had begun thinking about my departure from Saint Leo and was planning to retire in the Spring of 2021. My plan changed when the university sent the "senior faculty" of the university a voluntary offer to retire at the end of 2019 (retirement option). I initially ignored the offer of the retirement option until I reread the document and discussed it with my family, my attorney, and my financial planner. I accepted the retirement option and left Saint Leo in December. I was looking forward to retirement and new opportunities and adventures like more time on the golf course, biking, and travel. What awaited me was certainly not what I expected as I found myself embarking on my reluctant journey as a cancer patient; in my case it was prostate cancer.

In mid-December of 2019, after cleaning out my office at the university, I traveled with my wife to visit the Cleveland Clinic in Palm Beach. I was having trouble sleeping and was experiencing recurring pain in my upper extremities and in my lower back. I met with the nurse practitioner who ordered a set of x-rays for my back and a PSA test. (PSA stands for protein-specific antigen. It is a blood test that indicates the level of a specific protein and is usually the first test given to detect the possible presence of prostate cancer.) I was a little surprised by the choice of the PSA test as my regular physician visits in Tampa in recent years indicated satisfactory or good levels for all the "regular" tests. I assumed that included the PSA test. I was amazed to learn that the PSA test results were not included in the records of my regular tests. A few days into the new year, I received the test results from the Clinic: degenerating discs in my lower back, evidence of scoliosis and an extremely high PSA result (over 39). I was shocked. Actually, I felt like I had been hit by a ton of bricks. How could this happen?

After receiving the news of my high PSA number, I contacted Dr. Patrick Walsh, former director of the James Brady Urological Institute at Johns

Hopkins Medical School to discuss my situation. (My father was a urologist and endowed a scholarship for the urology program at Hopkins, his medical school alma mater so Dr. Walsh was my "go to" guy.) Dr. Walsh is the author of "Guide to Surviving Prostate Cancer" and is well known in the field of urology.

I had my copy of his book out and read as much as I could to better understand prostate cancer. My initial thought was to travel to Baltimore to meet with Dr. Walsh, with Dr. Alan Partin the current Director of the Brady, and other members of the urology staff at the Brady and have them do a thorough urological exam and then schedule a radical prostatectomy to remove the prostate and the cancer, if that proved to be the ultimate diagnosis.

My plan changed when he told me of a urologist in Tampa, Dr. David Hernandez who is a Brady graduate, and a very well-respected urologist in the Tampa Bay area at Tampa General Hospital (TGH). I met with Dr. Hernandez and he did another PSA test which was lower (a good sign) and a biopsy of the prostate. The diagnosis: stage 3 prostate cancer.

I was stunned by the news. There were no symptoms. How did this happen? Shock turned to shame and embarrassment. My father was a preeminent urologist who performed one of the earliest prostatectomies at University Hospitals in Cleveland and did some significant research in the area of prostate cancer. I thought I knew a lot about prostate cancer, but I never imagined it would happen to me. As the reality of the diagnosis set in, I felt a sense of fear as I tried to accept the reality that I was now a cancer patient.

Dr. Hernandez met with me and my wife in late January to discuss the "plan of attack" to beat the cancer. I have several friends who have had prostate cancer, and each chose a different approach to deal with the cancer: radical prostatectomy, radiation seeds implanted in the prostate and cryotherapy. Some have had a combination of all of the above. I originally planned to have a radical prostatectomy because I was not keen on having the seeds inserted into my prostate and being "radioactive." I ruled out cryotherapy as one of my friends who had gone the cryotherapy route lost control of his bladder.

The doctor described a different approach that we would follow to deal with the cancer. The treatment would be "external beam radiation therapy" (EBRT), considered by many in the urology field to be the new "gold standard" for treating prostate cancer. There would be no surgery or radiation seeds inserted into the prostate. My bone and CT scans showed the cancer had not spread outside the prostate. Still, there was one lymph node adjacent to the prostate that concerned him. With EBRT he would radiate the prostate, and the surrounding area where the lymph node was located, to kill the cancer. The treatment would also include hormone therapy (Androgen Deprivation Therapy or ADT) to remove testosterone to shrink the prostate and help prevent the cancer from returning after successful completion of the EBRT. ADT brings with it "night sweats" and frequent trips to the bathroom each night. (As I tell my friends, I am going through "manopause") This therapy also impacts the patient's muscle tone and overall strength, and it can negatively impact a patient's hip joints and/or lead to osteoporosis. I realized this one day as I was trying to pick up a box of some household items that did not appear to weigh much. I struggled to pick up the box and I later saw myself in the mirror and realized I now had "stick arms and legs" and had dropped approximately 25 pounds (I wanted to drop some weight, but not in this fashion). I was now at the lowest weight I had seen since my graduate school days at Florida State in the late 1970's.

As Dr. Lawrence Berk, who would be coordinating the radiation therapy, was setting up the schedule for my radiation treatments, everyone's world came to a halt with the COVID-19 pandemic. Just about everything in the Tampa Bay area shut down due to the virus in an effort to control it. I was extremely concerned. What did this mean for my cancer treatment? Hospitals canceled all "non-essential" or elective medical procedures and surgeries. Fortunately, EBRT to battle prostate cancer was considered an essential medical procedure and we moved forward with the treatment plan. I would have 25 radiation treatments over the course of 5 weeks. Before we could start the treatments, gold markers would be inserted into the prostate, but the delivery of the markers took longer than expected and that delayed the process a few weeks. I sat around waiting to get started, wondering how all this would play out.

The hormone therapy began with the first quarterly injection in early February and the radiation treatments began in late March. Each day, I would arrive at the TGH parking garage at approximately 9:40 a.m. and contact the Cancer Center from my cell phone. When they were ready for me, they would call me back and I would walk from the parking garage to the entrance of the Cancer Center. The staff met me at the door, took my temperature and gave me my patient bracelet for the day's treatment. Then, the radiation therapists (not technicians as they explained to me) met me and took me back for the day's treatments. They were always upbeat, and I tried to be the same, even though some days I was not "feeling it" but I usually greeted them with "Good morning ladies, let's go kill some cancer" and we all laughed. On more than one occasion, I heard them say that they wished more patients had the same attitude.

The therapists were always prepared and very efficient. We followed the same routine for each session. I would get on the table and they would put me in the "tube" (not an MRI tube, but a much shorter tube) to take a picture of my prostate to see how the radiation therapy was progressing in defeating the cancer. After a minute or two, they would put me back into the "tube" for the radiation therapy session. I was impressed with how precise they were in their observations. On at least two occasions, they informed me that my buttocks were not "relaxed", and they had to reposition me on the table. (I had never known I could "relax" my butt.) The radiation therapy process was painless, and I was pleasantly surprised at how brief the sessions were – usually 10 minutes. For each session, I was allowed to select the music of my choice and I usually selected classical music with the idea that it would relax me. Some days it worked well, on other days, not so much. I did not always get to pick the specific pieces that were played during my sessions. Trying to remain relaxed with Beethoven's 5th Symphony blaring in your ears was indeed a challenge!

While the sessions were brief and painless, they were fatiguing and took more out of me than I realized. There were many afternoon "siestas" while I would watch TV through my eyelids. I did my best each day to maintain an upbeat attitude as I went through the course of radiation therapy, but some days were better than others. I recall one afternoon when I had come back from TGH and I was not feeling my best. I was reading emails and one really struck me. The pandemic had shut down most of the nation, but a group of musicians had gotten together virtually and played "Ode to Joy" from Beethoven's 9th Symphony, one of my all-time classical favorites. The music struck just the right inner chord and I was reduced to tears, bawling like a little boy. I have continued to listen to classical music frequently over the weeks and months of this journey. Conductor-violinist Andre Rieu has become one of my favorites and I can listen to the music of his orchestra for hours on end and not tire of it. It is very moving and relaxing at the same time and the music fills my heart with hope, not just for my recovery, but for full recovery for others who are worse off than I am. I successfully completed the radiation therapy in late April without difficulty and my last two PSA test scores came back at under 0.1, which is essentially non-detectable.

NOT A CANCER PATIENT

By
Bonnie Cashin Farmer

When I was invited to be a contributor to this book publication, I replied that I did not belong among these courageous individuals living with cancer because "I am not a cancer patient". Admittedly in January 2015, I was diagnosed with Invasive Ductal Carcinoma (ID) Breast Cancer Stage 1A which required an immediate lumpectomy, radiation, plus an aromatase inhibitor medication for a minimum of five years. Under different circumstances, such news might have been more upsetting and frightening to me but instead this news created immediate fear of how I would be able to care for my spouse who, less than three months before, was diagnosed with aggressive multiple myeloma. At the time of my diagnosis, his pain was completely uncontrolled, his hospitalizations were numerous, and his health status was severely compromised and continuing to deteriorate. When the date of my previously scheduled annual routine mammogram was due, I had seriously considered cancelling my appointment. However, since we were at the hospital anyway, I fortunately decided to keep my appointment. As a registered nurse, I have always valued the importance of routine screenings; this time was no exception.

We all bring our own unique perspective of our experiences with cancer. Being a registered nurse remains embedded within who I am and informs every aspect of my being as a cancer patient and being a cancer caregiver. To this day my two adult children still tease me of always "assessing and evaluating" their wellness upon first greeting in a manner like a nurse's constant patient focus. Thus, my perspectives throughout these writings reflect the triple lens of cancer patient, cancer caregiver, and registered nurse.

My cancer diagnosis added another dimension of burden for our family already in crisis. I genuinely was not as upset with my diagnosis as one might think because I was so focused on my spouse and how to provide the intense care that he required. I was more annoyed than anything else because my cancer was interfering with caregiving. I proceeded with my cancer in a robotic manner: putting one foot in front of the other and addressing my cancer while at the same time navigating my spouse's tortuous condition. I considered my cancer to be insignificant as compared to my spouse's cancer. I shared my diagnosis with only my closest friends.

When I had my first visit with the oncologist, within the same oncology organization as my spouse, I made a mental comment that I am not like many of the other seriously ill patients in the waiting room; I was not ill, sick, nor compromised. While sitting next to a middle-aged couple holding hands with a patient wrist band visible on one hand, I also made another mental notation that from the very beginning I knew that I would be going this road alone. My spouse was critically ill and had little to no comprehension of my current condition. The licensed clinical social worker from "our" cancer office had gently approached me on several occasions during the first few months of my diagnosis and treatment to inquire if I would like to talk. I vehemently replied, "Oh no- I was doing just fine."

As a tenured professor of nursing, I reluctantly requested a Family Leave for the remainder of that spring semester. I commented that the human resource officer could take her pick of diagnoses for the paperwork. I returned to work late summer 2015. My spouse received a stem cell transplant in fall 2015 and I foolishly continued to work despite having additional earned Family Leave available. During his lengthy post-transplant hospitalization, I stayed at a nearby hotel that offered a daily shuttle to the hospital. I provided alternative arrangements for my students and made the four-hour round trip for a specific class only once during that time.

By December 2015, when an ordinary two-hour grading project took over ten hours, I recognized that "perhaps" I might need a "little" help and began to consider some professional counseling. I was disgusted with myself as I certainly knew all the answers (or so I thought at the time) yet did not have the capacity to implement some strategic stress reduction interventions on my own.

During my first counseling meeting, I truly forgot to share the fact of my diagnosis of breast cancer less than three months after my spouse's catastrophic diagnosis. Only as I was walking out the door after our one-hour appointment, I turned around and said, "Oh, I forgot to mention that I had breast cancer at the same time." My professional counselor has remained a much appreciated and important member of my current team. For a long time, I remained not a cancer patient.

Several years later, while sitting in the oncology waiting room with my spouse for his appointment, the staff receptionist called me over. She said that she had something for "me." She reached behind her desk for a lovely holiday gift: full of nail products including pretty polishes, nail files dotted with sparkles, and fun nail stickers. She told me that a volunteer had donated the gift for a cancer patient. As I was blankly staring, she said "well, you have several granddaughters, don't you?" I replied, "Yes, but I am not a cancer patient." She kindly looked at me and softly reminded me that I was a cancer patient. I gratefully received the gift set and began to quietly cry as I returned to my chair.

I have never been in denial regarding my cancer, but my primary focus has always been on my spouse's cancer. Genetic counseling at the time of my diagnosis revealed that I was a carrier of a genetic mutation that was related to breast cancer and colorectal cancer. Following the immediate interventions of surgery and radiation, I was prescribed an aromatase inhibitor, the preferred adjuvant treatment for post-menopausal women with estrogen receptor- positive breast cancer. With still more than three years left in my treatment plan, debilitating side effects to my hands required a change to a different aromatase inhibitor. As I contended with the oftentimes challenging side effects of any aromatase inhibitor, I looked forward to completion of the recommended five-year plan of medication treatment. With periodic physical screenings and yearly mammograms, I made another mental note to myself that I could and would do this.

In the latter fourth year of my aromatase inhibitor treatment, I began to experience unexplained weight loss. At first, I was unconcerned. I was maintaining a life-long healthy diet combined with both formal and informal exercise. Since losing weight without trying was a novel experience for me, I admittedly was pleased until the scale kept going down. For my entire life, I had never lost weight without being very deliberate with much effort and sometimes with little success. During non-cancer related routine medical follow-ups, medical professionals noted the then five-to-ten-pound loss as probably being stress- related. During a routine appointment with my oncologist, I casually asked what my weight had been since my last visit. I had lost twenty pounds. Her concern was evident. This was the very first time that the words metastases and me were used in the same sentence. For all my knowledge and understanding of breast cancer, I was numb to hear that my "creepy-crawly" cancer could metastasize. "Creepy-crawly" was the actual description from the radiologist at the time of diagnosis. Prior to that day, I had never given earnest consideration for other developing cancers within my body.

For the next two months a series of comprehensive imaging, screening, and testing revealed some identified areas for increased surveillance and no malignancies. My health status for establishment of a surveillance risk plan was further complicated by the absence of familial hereditary information. I entered this world through a Salvation Army birth supported program and adopted by my beloved parents at the age of six months. Since early childhood, my adoption was a known fact to me. Upon the birth of my children, my parents gave the original birth certificate to me. An additional shred of health information verbally emerged at that time: cancer.

This next to almost non-existent knowledge of familial hereditary cancer has proven a considerable factor in establishing my plan of treatment and surveillance post five years treatment. After reaching the five-year mark of medication in spring of 2020, an appointment with my oncologist focused on the benefits and risks of continuing aromatase inhibitor treatment. Since my spouse was doing just "okay," I requested to postpone this important and complicated decision. My oncologist agreed. With compassionate and competent counsel from my oncologist, we decided to continue the medication until the following fall.

I then requested a follow up meeting with genetic counseling. The genetic counselor had advised me to check with them as needed for any new findings, updates, and changes in the evidence/research that might impact my future health decisions and protocol. The genetic counselor informed me that, in 2019, evidence of new research determined my genetic mutation not to be related to breast cancer: only to colorectal cancer. For an instant I thought good-bye to the aromatase inhibitor! The genetic counselor quickly highlighted the scant knowledge of familial hereditary cancer accompanied by no knowledge of any familial health: translated my potential risk for breast cancer remains.

Subsequent surveillance for colorectal cancer also required additional due diligence on my part. Much of the established gastrointestinal protocols for surveillance risk are framed within the context of familial hereditary health and disease history. I requested a follow-up appointment with my gastrointestinal physician. Upon further discussion of my request for increased gastrointestinal surveillance, given my current health status and absence of familial history, he did acknowledge that few formal protocols include individuals with my gene mutation, gastrointestinal health history, and absence of familial hereditary history. We then established a revised plan of surveillance.

In late fall 2020, my oncologist and I created a plan of continued aromatase inhibitor treatment until the time of my upcoming mammogram and a bone density test two weeks later followed by an oncology appointment for treatment assessment. In some respects, I feel more like a cancer patient today than ever before; thoughts of metastases now linger around in the back of my head.

The absence of knowledge for familial hereditary cancers forces my hand for due diligence. I feel an intense obligation to my spouse and my family to leave no stone unturned in seeking and maintaining my care. Making emotional room for my cancer, related treatments, and vigilant surveillance still seem burdensome at best. Yet perhaps the time has come for me to revisit "I am not a cancer patient."

THOSE THREE WORDS

By
Cherie LaFlamme Genua

The year leading up to my cancer diagnosis was—in one word—busy. Between finishing my MBA, planning a wedding, and selling and buying a house, I did not have a spare moment. It is no wonder that I ignored the lump in my left breast for so long. I first noticed it the summer before my diagnosis. I was standing in the shower at my in-law's home, which is where we were living while we waited for our house to be ready. I rubbed against the lump, figuring it was a cyst. I dismissed it. From time-to-time, I would reach down my shirt and touch it, never once thinking it was anything more than dense breast tissue or something benign. However, it was when the lump started growing over the months that I knew something was wrong. I contacted my primary care doctor and made an appointment.

I canceled my first appointment in September. I claimed that the timing did not work with my meeting schedule at my new job. That is what I told myself, anyway—but in reality, I was terrified. Another month went by and the internal alarms rang. I was driving home from work and received a phone call about a relative who was diagnosed with an aggressive form of glioblastoma. That phone call changed my life. I was horrified for my family member and what he was dealing with as he received treatment and fought for his life. I vowed to go see my doctor once and for all. "What the hell am I waiting for?" I asked myself before sneaking into a supply closet at work to make the appointment. No one else was going to prioritize my health—it was up to me.

A few days later, I sat on the cold table of my primary care physician's office in a johnny-coat as he felt my left breast. He felt the lump right away without any direction. In the next breath, he ordered an emergency mammogram and ultrasound. It is probably a good time to mention that I was 34 at the time and a regular screening would not have come until 6 years later had I not felt the lump on my own. I left his office and within minutes, the mammogram scheduler called me and asked me to come in. "Can you be here in thirty minutes?" she asked. I dropped everything—including the iced coffee I was drinking, which went all over my car—and drove to the hospital.

The mammogram and ultrasound were painless, of course, but that did not stop my heart from racing. The ultrasound technician finished and had the radiologist review my reports immediately. He walked in and sat down in front of me. "This looks like a suspicious mass to me," he said. "I have already scheduled a biopsy for you for the breast and under the arm. We will get you an appointment with the breast surgeons as well to go over your results."

I left that office in a panic and sat in my car in the parking lot. The first call I made was to my new boss of only two months. He could barely understand me through the sobbing, but there was no way I could come into work in that condition. I went home and tried my best to distract myself. I knew the mass was not a cyst and that there was reason for concern, but I tried to hold it together until my biopsy appointment two days later.

The biopsy was performed on Thanksgiving Eve, which meant I had to wait the weekend before hearing the results. On Monday morning—exactly one year and one day after my wedding—my husband and I went to the breast surgeon's office. She walked in and laid it out with those three words you never want to hear: "You have cancer." The biopsy confirmed that it was, in fact, breast cancer and that it had spread to two lymph nodes that were also biopsied. "You are going to need chemo," she continued. I held it together until she said those few words. For some reason, I had not thought about needing chemotherapy until this point.

That night at home, I did my best to digest the news of my new diagnosis. Questions raced through my mind as I replayed my breast surgeons' conversation in my head. Why was this happening to me? How am I going to tell my family and friends? Would I be able to work through treatment? Would we be able to afford the new house we just bought? Was I going to lose my hair? How about my eyebrows? And of course: was I going to live or die? The truth is that getting diagnosed with cancer hits you like a ton of bricks, but the diagnosis is only the tip of the iceberg.

The week that followed my initial diagnosis was filled to the brim with tests—a breast MRI, a CT scan, bloodwork, and a PET scan (nuclear medicine). They were looking to see if my cancer had spread. I cried whenever a nurse, radiology tech, or phlebotomist asked me any question about my diagnosis. I recall sitting on a cold table in the hospital as I prepared for a CT scan. The nurse asked me a question unrelated to my diagnosis, but it still led to uncontrollable sobbing. She hugged me for as long as I let her and told me about her mother who was a breast cancer survivor well into her 80s. I connected with a lot of strangers that week. They helped me feel less alone as I navigated in and out of hospitals, radiology departments, and offices. I will never forget their kindness. Waiting for the results from these sets of tests was much harder than the initial biopsy results, and my breast surgeon knew it. As soon as she walked into the patient room she said, "the cancer did not spread." I nearly vomited in my lap. She made me an appointment with an oncologist to start discussing my treatment plan. I was ready to move forward. I was ready to put on a brave face and start treatment.

When my husband and I met with the oncologist, he laid out the plan. I was going to get a port-a-cath (port) placed, complete 16 rounds of chemotherapy over 20 weeks first to stop any further spread, then have surgery followed by radiation. In the meeting, he asked if we had children. "Not yet," I said, "but we were planning on it."

This development delayed the onset of my treatment by a few weeks. My oncologist said that preserving and harvesting my eggs was important before beginning chemotherapy if I wanted children of my own eventually. Time was of the essence, though, because my oncologist wanted to start chemotherapy immediately. I met with a leading endocrinologist two days later and started fertility treatments right away. In between other appointments and work meetings, I was at the fertility center every other day for bloodwork and ultrasounds to see how my eggs were progressing after the onslaught of hormone injections. I even gave myself a hormone injection in the bathroom at work one time as I cried out of stress and frustration (do you sense a theme here? The crying eased with time, thankfully). Two weeks later, on Christmas Eve, my sister-in-law gave me the trigger hormone injection. I had bloodwork on Christmas Day at an empty hospital, and my eggs were harvested promptly on the morning of

December 26th. I had 22 viable eggs that are still safely frozen in the fertility clinic waiting for my return.

Okay, now I was really ready.

My first chemotherapy infusion was one week later. I woke up early that morning, showered, and got dressed. I applied a numbing cream to my port site to ease my fear of the needle accessing my port (highly recommended, by the way—ask your oncologist about it!). I packed my chemo bag with magazines, snacks, calming coloring books, nausea lozenges, and headphones—and did not use any of it. Although I went through a thorough chemo education course with my oncology nurses, which taught me about side effects and how to manage them, it did not prepare me for how the actual chemotherapy would feel as it went into my body. My senses were heightened as I sat through my first infusion of the drugs doxorubicin hydrochloride (Adriamycin) and cyclophosphamide. Adriamycin is known in the breast cancer community as "the red devil" because the drug is administered from a large syringe containing red liquid and is injected intravenously. Aside from the color, it puts you out. But for a great reason—it works hard to destroy cancer cells in your body. I sat in the chemo room for about six hours as the drugs dripped into my body. I did not feel much, to be honest. These days, the nurses premedicate with medication that helps fight off the rough side effects. I can still taste the anti-nausea drugs that were pumped through my port somehow, but they were lifesavers because my nausea mostly subsided throughout treatment. My mom and husband sat by my side that day and kept me company, which is why I never needed the contents of my chemo bag to entertain me.

One misconception people have about chemotherapy is that it takes place in a gloomy environment where everyone dwelled about being sick. My experience was far different. The nurses were all comforting and upbeat, and you become friends with your fellow patients in neighboring recliners. The space was bright and exuded positivity. It was lively depending on the day, there was a volunteer hand masseuse or a guitarist softly strumming songs in the background. Yes, some patients are quite sick—but the feeling you get when you walk through the door was "hope" not fear. Definitely not death. Everyone is there to fight and to forge ahead, no matter what the outcome might be. There is a camaraderie in a cancer center that is like no other.

It's difficult to sugarcoat the days following chemotherapy, though, although everyone's experiences are wildly different. I was not nauseous, but I was tired. Think of a day in your life when fatigue took over—maybe after working a double shift or exploring a new city on foot over 20,000 steps. Now multiply that feeling by fifty. And add extreme bone pain and mental fog to the mix. But the good news in my situation was that the good days outweighed the bad. I often felt bad for a few days following chemo and then went back to feeling like my normal self until my next treatment.

I lived life as normally as possible working, cleaning my house, going out to dinner, and visiting with family and friends. I maintained a positive and gracious attitude throughout the good and bad days. Chemo did not destroy me and it was nothing to fear, after all. After 20 weeks, I rang the bell to indicate the end of chemotherapy as my family, oncologist, nurses, and staff rallied around me to celebrate. I rang that bell again at the end of immunotherapy and once more at the end of radiation. It might feel silly, but celebrating every win is an important part of a cancer journey. Every cheer, every flower, every gift—it all makes a difference in your attitude and your willingness to move forward.

A month after chemotherapy ended, I had breast surgery which also included pathology testing to show how effective chemo was in destroying my cancer cells. A few days after surgery, my plastic surgeon gave me a sneak peek of my pathology report. It showed that there was no evidence of disease in my breast or any of the lymph nodes that were tested. I could hardly believe it, but my breast surgeon and oncologist confirmed the great news with me as well. Chemo was a long and challenging road, but having clear pathology reports made all of the tears and pain worth it. Not everyone has this outcome, though, which is where your support system comes into play. They are an important part of your cancer journey and will play a huge role—no matter your age, stage, or prognosis.

After a strenuous fifteen months of treatment—including chemotherapy, surgery, radiation, and immunotherapy—I learned that the toughest part of my journey had not yet begun. During cancer treatment, I had an overwhelming feeling that I was "doing something" about the cancer in the hopes of destroying it. I went through the motions and fought cancer, as everyone so aptly wants you to do. On the last day of immunotherapy (the last phase of my specific treatment plan), my oncologist told me he would see me in three months. I felt like I was once again hit with a pile of bricks. Without the reassurance of regular blood work and check-ups, how could I possibly make it through each week and each day?

The end of treatment is a strange feeling. For starters, it is exciting—I got to ring the bell! I did not have to get poked so often! But, for me, it was also a lonely, scary, and emotionally draining time. "After Cancer" is not something that is talked about often enough. It was the time after treatment came to an end (for those in remission) where I no longer had to see my oncologist every few weeks. This is when my mind began to wander. Is the pain in my hip from my outdoor run a few days ago—or did the cancer return? Is this dry cough a cold—or did the cancer return? Is the fogginess I'm experiencing in my head months after treatment normal—or did the cancer return? Did this bruise on my leg happen after I hit my leg on the counter—or did the cancer return? You get the idea. These are all actual thoughts that ran, and still run, through my mind whenever something feels off in my body. I am able to work through some fears myself, while other aches and pains might require the assurance of a scan, x-ray, or bloodwork to put my mind at ease.

The fear of recurrence is something I have to work through every single day. This feeling never goes away, but I know it gets better with time. For me, the further I get away from treatment, the less I think about cancer. It no longer takes over my mind dozens of times an hour; instead, it rears its ugly head a few times a day. It will always be with me, but I will not let it define me. Cancer is life-changing, but I am more than cancer. I am a woman full of life and laughter—I love better, and I listen more. I am a woman who will not be debilitated by my thoughts or fears. And I am a woman who has changed for the better because of, and despite, my diagnosis. For that, I am grateful and hopeful.

DILEMMAS, DECISIONS, AND BEING A CANCER PATIENT

By
Burt Harres

My oldest son, Michael, served in the United States Marine Corps. He was assigned to the 1st Battalion, 6th Marines, Bravo Company based in Camp Lejeune, North Carolina. He was actively engaged in combat in Fallujah and Ar Ramadi, Iraq. I was single during his deployments and spent many sleepless nights, sitting in my leather recliner, praying that he and his fellow Marines would safely make it through the perils of war. I remember that one night, I prayed to God that if it was His will, to take my life to spare Michael's. I imagine my prayer was no different than that of countless parents whose prayers were like mine. As a Roman Catholic, I also knew that it is not appropriate to bargain with God, but fear has an incredible way of clouding our thoughts and misleading our actions. After that night, instead of bargaining with God, I was direct and simply asked him to keep Michael safe and to bring him home alive. God more than answered my prayers. Michael returned home. You might be asking yourself, what does my son's service in the Marine Corps have to do with my being a cancer patient? I will answer this question in a few paragraphs.

Years ago, when I reached my "Big Five O" (50th) birthday, I begrudgingly accepted the realization that physical exams would become part of my life's annual rituals. When I was a kid, I had to get an annual physical exam to participate in my school's athletic programs, particularly baseball and basketball: No big deal. I would schedule an appointment with our family doctor, show up, he would take my temperature, ask me to cough, check my glands, listen to my heart, and had me "drop trou" (pull down my pants and check that my private parts were in order). Then he would sign the participation form, I would pay $2.00 for the visit, and I was on my way.

Well, the years have passed by quickly and now I approach my annual physical exam with a bit of trepidation. Are the little aches and pains I experience merely a sign of getting older or is something seriously transpiring? Fortunately, I have a wonderful family medical physician who helps answer this question.

"Dr. Bob," as I admirably and respectfully call him, and I have quite a history. Before he begins my annual physical exam, we talk about current events, provide updates on mutual friends, and tell jokes. I recall years ago he was digitally checking my prostate while simultaneously telling a joke. We were laughing hysterically when his nurse opened the door to give him a message. The look on her face when she saw us laughing while "Dr. Bob" had his finger in my rectum to check my prostate was priceless.

Fast forward to 2012, "Dr. Bob" was once again checking my prostate. But this time, there was no laughter. He was deadly serious. He said he felt something odd. He told me that I might have an enlarged prostate but just to be sure of my condition, he recommended a urologist for follow-up. Little did I know that from this appointment I was about to embark on a life-altering journey.

During my initial meeting with the urologist, he described the process he would follow when performing the biopsy of my prostate. A prostate biopsy is usually performed using a transrectal ultrasound (TRUS). The images taken with the ultrasound help the urologist guide a fine needle to the areas selected for sampling. The spring-loaded needle is attached to the ultrasound probe and enters the prostate through the rectum. There is some pressure felt by the patient when the probe is inserted, but it is usually not painful. Usually, six to ten prostatic tissue samples are taken. The procedure takes approximately ten minutes. The prostatic tissue samples are examined by a pathologist to determine whether cancer or other abnormal cells are in the prostate gland. The pathologist sends a report to the doctor who then provides the results of the pathologist's findings to the patient.

When my urologist described the prostate biopsy procedure to me, my skin became clammy. I am convinced that when it comes to discussing prostate biopsies, the male gender and I are on the top of the list for being reduced to a pile of wimps. Nevertheless, I knew I had to proceed with the biopsy, so I scheduled an appointment for the procedure.

When my urologist performed the biopsy of my prostate, the procedure went according to plan. I felt minor discomfort when he biopsied six tissues and the procedure was over in less than fifteen minutes. He told me he would have the results in seven to ten days. I was relieved that the procedure was over, but still anxious about what the results would reveal.

Tuesday, October 30, 2012, was a beautiful sunny day as well as my granddaughter's first birthday. I also anticipated hearing from my urologist sometime this week. As Vice President of Instruction/Provost at a local community college, I went into work as usual. My day at work was typical and I remember having lunch with my staff in our conference room when my administrative assistant informed me that I had an important phone call on hold. When I picked up the phone, my urologist's nurse said the pathologist's report had arrived and that my urologist wanted to see me. My immediate response was that I would be in his office in 30 minutes. Fortunately, my schedule for the afternoon was open. I told my administrative assistant that I needed to leave campus and see my doctor.

The normal 30-minute drive to my urologist's office seemed like an eternity. Upon arrival, I checked my watch to note the drive had been completed in about 20 minutes. When I entered the doctor's office, the nurse seemed surprised. She said that I hung up before she could schedule an appointment for me to see the urologist and that his afternoon was booked seeing patients. I was embarrassed that I had let fear overcome me and sheepishly asked that if I waited, would the doctor see me after he saw his last scheduled patient. She checked with the doctor and returned with an affirmative response. The next two hours passed as if they were two days. I recall paging through old magazines, not really reading them, but simply trying to keep my mind occupied. Finally, around four o'clock, the urologist appeared and asked me to follow him into his office.

I am rather good at reading body language so as we sat down in my urologist's office, I sensed that I was in store for some bad news. My intuition was correct. The pathologist's report indicated that two of the six prostatic tissues indicated cell abnormalities that were a sign of prostate cancer. The results from a prostate biopsy are usually given in the form of a Gleason score. On the simplest level, the scoring system assigns a number from 2 to 10 to describe the abnormal cells. The lower the Gleason score, the less likely the cancer is going to spread to the lymph nodes, bones, or other organs. My Gleason score was 3+4=7 which is considered a medium-grade cancer. The 3 represented the largest area of the tumor and the 4 described the cells of the second largest area. I learned that tumors with a primary score of 3 and a secondary score of 4 have a fairly good outlook. So, despite the gloomy news, there was somewhat of a "silver lining" in the pathologist's report.

My urologist and I discussed potential treatment plans. He suggested that I seriously consider prostate cancer robotic assisted surgery with da Vinci technology to remove my prostate gland. We discussed the pros and cons of this type of treatment. He provided me with material about this procedure and the telephone number of a surgeon in Orlando, Florida who is nationally recognized for performing radical prostatectomies with da Vinci technology. My urologist asked me to think about what I would like to do, talk to the surgeon, and get back with him in a week or two with my decision. My urologist also ordered several tests including an intravenous pyelogram, whole bone body scan, and chest x-ray. As I left my urologist's office, I recall that thousands of thoughts flooded my mind. One of them was the prayer I made to God years before when my son, Michael, was engaged in combat in Iraq. I thought, well maybe it is God's will that Michael's life would be spared in place of mine. But again, I quickly realized that, as a Roman Catholic, we are taught and believe that God does not work that way. However, I later learned that the thoughts I experienced are normal.

When we receive bad news, we encounter grief with its wide variety of emotions such as sorrow, misery, anguish, pain, annoyance, and sadness. Grief is universal and very personal. When one experiences grief, crying, becoming angry, withdrawing from others, and feeling empty are common reactions. None of these are unusual or wrong. Everyone grieves differently, but there are some commonalities in the stages and feelings experienced during grief. Dr. Elisabeth Kubler-Ross developed a theory of the five stages of grief, also known as the "Kubler-Ross Model" which was originally designed for people who were ill. The five stages of grief are: denial, anger, bargaining, depression, and acceptance. Not everyone will experience all five stages, and a person may not go through them in this order. In my case, during my concern about Michael's safety and again when I received the bad results about my prostate biopsy, I was in the bargaining stage of grief. Kubler-Ross explained that during the bargaining stage, a person feels vulnerable and helpless. It is common that when a person is in the bargaining stage of grief that they look for ways to regain control or find ways to affect the outcome of an event. Kubler-Ross also asserted that it is common for religious individuals to make a deal or promise to God, or a higher power, in return for relief from the grief and/or healing. The research conducted by Kubler-Ross helped me understand why I entered the bargaining stage of grief and explained why I was able to better embrace the acceptance stage when I was diagnosed with having prostate cancer.

At this point in my journey as a cancer patient, I offer my first set of take-aways:

- Schedule and keep, do not postpone, annual check-ups with your doctor.
- Do not delay in following up with your doctor's recommendations.
- If the results of tests/biopsies do not come back with good news, the experience of grief is perfectly normal.

After meeting with my urologist and receiving the results of the pathologist's report, I spent a great deal of time researching the treatment option that he suggested. By November 6, 2012, I completed the recommended tests. However, I was not completely sold on the idea of having a radical prostatectomy. I recalled that a former colleague of mine was diagnosed with prostate cancer and had positively commented on the expert medical care and treatment that he received. I called my friend, explained my situation, and sought his advice. He highly recommended that I request a consultation with Michael Dattoli, MD, physician-in-chief/board certified radiation oncologist at the Dattoli Cancer Center and Brachytherapy Research Institute in Florida. This oncologist, with over two decades of brachytherapy experience, is considered a foremost pioneer in brachytherapy designs that maximize tumor eradication and minimize symptoms. Furthermore, my colleague insisted that I not decide on how I would proceed with my prostate cancer treatment until such consultation. Valuing his opinion, I promised him I would follow his advice.

By late November, via a scheduled telephone call, my soon-to-be radiation oncologist and I discussed my condition for almost one hour. As I listened intently, I was extremely impressed with his expertise, compassion, and approach to treating prostate cancer. Brachytherapy, one type of radiation therapy to treat cancer, is a procedure that involves placing radioactive material inside your body. Brachytherapy allows doctors to deliver higher doses of radiation to more-specific areas of the body, compared with the conventional form of radiation therapy (external beam radiation) that projects radiation from a machine outside of your body. Brachytherapy may cause fewer side effects than external beam radiation, and the overall treatment time is usually shorter. After a restless night's sleep in which I must have been subconsciously wrestling with what I should do, I decided to secure brachytherapy treatment for my prostate cancer. I will be forever grateful to my colleague for recommending additional consultation for treatment options with his oncologist before making a final decision regarding my prostate cancer treatment.

Following my telephone consultation with the oncologist, I met with my urologist and informed him that I decided to receive prostate cancer treatment in lieu of the radical prostatectomy with da Vinci technology. He seemed disappointed in my decision and encouraged me to reconsider. Nevertheless, I stood by my decision and he accepted it with reservations. I asked, and he complied, with my request to send a copy of my medical file to the radiation oncologist.

The following narrative briefly summarizes the protocols and treatment plan I received. It is important to note that these protocols and treatment plan were recommended in November 2012 and may or may not be current as of the time of this writing.

Prior to my formal consultation with the radiation oncologist, I was required to obtain:

- A comprehensive bloodwork to include a PSA (prostate-specific antigen), percent free PSA, PAP (prostatic acid phosphatase), IGF-1, testosterone panel (including a total and bio- available testosterone, sex hormone binding globulin, DHEAS, DHT, androstenedione, prolactin LH, estradiol), LDH, vitamin D 1 and 25, D 25- hydroxy, vitamin B 12, folate, N-telopeptide, crosslinked, PTH (parathyroid hormone), calcitonin, osteocalcin, and urinalysis with cytology.
- A dynamic contrast enhanced pelvic/prostate MRI to further evaluate the cancer within the prostate, the integrity of the prostate capsule, status of seminal vesicles, and neurovascular bundles.

I was also required to provide all my urologist's relevant medical records including the biopsy report and the actual prostate biopsy slides, laboratory results, x-ray/scan reports, physician office notes, ultrasound reports, procedure notes. My most recent EKG and colonoscopy reports from "Dr. Bob" were also obtained for this comprehensive prior record review.

My formal consultation with the radiation oncologist included:

- 3D color flow Doppler ultrasound with penile vascular imaging.
- Bone mineral densitometry scan (QCT scan) to evaluate bone density and risk of osteoporosis.
- Fine section (2mm) helical CT scans of the chest/abdomen/pelvis for the purpose of determining any anatomical treatment related considerations.

My initial and formal consultations with the radiation oncologist further strengthened my confidence in my decision to have him and his staff treat my prostate cancer. His treatment protocol for me consisted of an attenuated course of DART (dynamic adaptive radiation therapy using four-dimensional guided intensity modulated external beam techniques) delivered over a period of 30 days preceding a seeding procedure. I began the DART treatment on December 24, 2012, and completed this procedure on February 5, 2013.

After I completed the DART treatment, there was a 43-day break between the completion of the DART and seeding procedure. Prior to the seeding procedure, on March 21, 2013, the radiation oncologist had his staff physicist perform a dose analysis of all prostate and periprostatic tissue. I was then required to stay in the hospital overnight following the seeding procedure.

I did not experience any discomfort from the daily DART treatment and the seeding procedure. The only pain I experienced was when the catheter that was inserted after the seeding procedure became blocked. The nurse temporarily removed the catheter in the middle of the night to evacuate the blockage. To my surprise, the second the catheter was removed, I was relieved of the discomfort but also urinated as if my penis was a foundation. I was terribly embarrassed but comforted when the nurse said that my situation was a common occurrence for patients after a seeding procedure. Despite her comforting words, my son, David, and I slid out of the hospital like thieves in the night when I was discharged at 5:00 a.m. on March 22, 2013. I would be remiss if I did not mention how helpful and supportive David was throughout my treatment process, and especially during my hospital stay.

On March 22, 2013, I had an appointment with my radiation oncologist so that he could determine the status of my condition after the seeding procedure. My examination went well, and I was told to rest for the rest of the day and then resume my normal activities. On June 20, 2013, I began a post-seeding boost treatment. Radiation therapy following the seed implant is known as a post-seeding boost. This treatment boosts the dose of radiation to specific sites to optimally kill microscopic cancer cells which may be present in the surrounding tissue. This course of therapy required a new CAT scan (Computed Technology Scan) because the dosimetry staff needs to use the results of the CAT scan to prepare an updated treatment plan.

On June 20, 2013, I began the daily post-seeding boost treatment that was completed on June 28, 2013, the day before my 61st birthday.

I continue to have annual follow-up examinations with the radiation oncologist. These follow-up visits include a review of my bloodwork, 3D color flow Doppler ultrasound, and CT scans of my lungs, prostate, and pelvic areas. As of this writing, I have been in remission for almost eight years. At this point in my journey as a cancer patient, I offer this second set of take-aways:

- If possible, do not rush into deciding your cancer treatment. A full range of treatment options for prostate cancer exist depending upon many factors for consideration. Try to become familiar with potential treatments so that you can better understand and discuss these various treatment options with your doctor. For example, according to the Mayo Clinic, a low-grade prostate cancer may not need treatment right away; doctors sometimes recommend active surveillance. Also, surgery might be a feasible option for treating cancer that is confined to the prostate; or used to treat advanced prostate cancer in combination with other treatments.

- Radiation therapy involves radiation that comes from outside one's body (external beam radiation). The patient lies on a table while a machine moves around his body, directing high-powered energy beams to the prostate cancer. Brachytherapy is a form of radiation treatment that involves placing radioactive sources in one's prostate tissue within the body. Ablative therapies can be used for prostate cancer by destroying prostate tissue with cold or heat. Hormone therapy is a treatment to stop a man's body from producing testosterone which may cause cancer cells to die or grow more slowly. Chemotherapy treatment is used to kill rapidly growing cells, including cancer cells. Immunotherapy uses one's immune system to fight cancer. I believe there is a natural tendency among many men to want to have the cancer treated immediately in the most expeditious manner. However, once a man decides on that type of prostate treatment he wants to receive, it is often difficult or impossible to change treatments once the process is initiated. More in-depth description of these prostate cancer treatment options can be found on the Mayo Clinic Prostate Cancer website.
- Do not be reluctant to obtain a second opinion from a different doctor and talk to men who have undergone prostate cancer treatment. Many doctors have their preferred treatment for prostate cancer which may or may not be the best option for the patient. A man can gain valuable information and insights by talking to other men who are currently receiving or previously received prostate cancer treatments.

For me, being a cancer patient involves experiencing the dilemmas of treatment options available for my prostate cancer and making the best personal treatment decisions.

CHAPTER TWO:

OBTAINING SUPPORT

STRESS AND SUPPORT GROUPS

By
Richard E. Farmer

My teaching experiences quickly became devoted to helping students learn the knowledge and details of their new academic major and eventually a career. As time went on, another psychology colleague of mine worked with me to create a model to help us, and clients, better understand people's experiences, both working on the job, and off. Called "The Stress Behavior Model," it is designed to help people to comprehend the role that stress plays in their behavior and their lives in general. It is important to point out that the concept of stress clearly includes any and all cancer diagnoses.

So, the idea or concept behind the Stress Behavior Model is to help individuals to understand the idea that all of us experience sources of stress which come as part of our daily living including family, friends, work colleagues, and our reactions to day-to-day living and working. These experiences can be both universal in that virtually all of us experience the same or similar things, or highly unique often as a result of our own personalities. These experiences create a very wide range of feelings in us that force us to behave in ways which allow us to cope, understand, or eliminate the feelings or the sources. The important point here is to understand that the behaviors we choose have either negative or positive consequences in the context for us as individuals or as members of one type of group or another.

Even though we may not have thought of it as such, all of us have participated in groups that could be considered as support groups. When we were younger, these groups were our friends, our teammates, fellow classmates, dorm roommates, co-workers and colleagues, spouses and families, children especially as we age, sports buddies, neighbors, clubs, or other recreational groups and/or religious organizations that we belong to. The idea is that all of us have connections with other people and these connections are sources of information about how to act with good or bad consequences. Learning how to act given a particular set of circumstances is fundamental to our human experience. And as we all know, the "how to act" of our behavior can be an additional source of stressors. So, our current understanding of behavior may well suggest that we "learn" behaviors that have positive or negative consequences for us. The idea here is that we have to be careful with the behaviors that we use to cope with various sources of stress. This is to suggest that all behaviors have consequences, good or bad, positive, or negative that will help us to cope. What we must avoid are coping behaviors which in and of themselves can become additional sources of stress and for obvious reasons.

In general, there are both formal and informal support groups. Informal groups come from our associations with friends, colleagues, neighbors, and the like. They just sort of happen because of our relationship with the individuals involved. Formal groups are deliberate, and people join because they wish to meet others with the same or similar interests, issues, or problems to solve. And, in the process of meeting and interacting, we learn how others may also be experiencing similar situations and how they use coping behaviors to deal with their experiences. This simply means that there is a "reason" that you are drawn to the set of individuals. Commonly, this reason is based on the purpose of the group's existence that we find attractive or the process of meeting that the group uses, and you find it acceptable. Finally, the known or assumed outcome of group belongingness is that we feel that the association could work for us.

Having been diagnosed with Multiple Myeloma more than five years ago, I decided that one of the things that I could do to remain engaged and stay active and positive was to help others in a similar situation. As one of the former coordinators of a blood cancers support group, I have once again been reminded of the power of being a member of a peer support group with a focused, shared experience. At the start, we are attracted to certain groups because of a particular purpose of that group. Unlike recreational, cultural, or neighborly groups, peer moderated support groups are almost always problem focused. Since we are experiencing a particular issue in our life, we seek out others who are also experiencing the same or similar problems. Thus, there is a sense of "mutuality" that draws us to one group or another. And this mutuality is how a group can provide support to its members since both moderators and participants share a similar experience and can readily learn from one another. What we have all seen is the commonality of the life-work experience which draws us to others because of the commonality of like experience or set of experiences.

You are strongly urged to look for a support group. This is based on the quite simple idea that these groups are a rich source of information about how others deal with the same or similar sources of stress that you are experiencing. This is to say that we have a lot to learn about our own current and future behavior by learning how others cope. As you look for a support group you need to pay attention to several principals. First, your potential support group should be regularly coming together addressing the same or similar problem(s) or sources that you are experiencing. And in the process of coming together it is important for you to assess and evaluate the "process" of support used by the members. For example, if one group you are interested in meets at a local establishment where alcohol flows plentifully, the obvious potential consequences that are legal, familial, or reputational become apparent. The obvious point to be made is that you need to exercise some degree of commonsense such that the support group itself does not become yet another source of negative or harmful stress. The process of deciding to join with a group that meets at a local bar or the health fitness center should be obvious.

While the overriding issue of cancer does bind all cancer patients together, the richness and utility of the support group that is specifically aimed at the problem one is encountering is best seen when members have as many details in common as possible, keeping in mind that diseases often express themselves differently to patients, caregivers, and families. The second and exceptionally important element of the support group is that the process of members supporting each other are doing so utilizing processes that are in and of themselves not problematic or do not run the risk of creating additional issues for you.

So, in deciding about which group or groups are available to provide you support, it is important for you to try to determine what you are looking for support for. It is imperative that you must come to terms with the idea that a cancer diagnosis in and of itself is a major source of stress. Clearly and virtually every aspect of our life is affected: Spouses, children, other family members, work, health care finances, ability to seek competent treatment, neighbors' religious organizations, self-concept, hobbies, personal attributes, ability to sustain intimacy, and the willingness to talk to others about your experiences with the disease.

SUPPORT

By
David W. Persky

Upon receiving my cancer diagnosis, I wondered what to do next. Was there a local prostate cancer support group in Tampa? Where would I find such a group? Fortunately, I did not need to look too far for support. My wife Mary and daughter Abigail have provided love and support for me every step of the way since I received my diagnosis. Mary is an HR professional, and she put her career search on hold so she could be with me during each leg of the journey. Abigail, one of the many furloughed staff members at Disney, came home from Orlando to pitch in and help in any way she could. When I began the radiation therapy at TGH (Tampa General Hospital), we developed a routine for each day's visit to the TGH Cancer Center. We would stop at Dunkin' Donuts each morning and get a donut (our Dunkin' fix) and something to drink for the short drive to TGH. When we got to the TGH parking garage, I would check in at the Cancer Center. Mary would catch up with friends on social media or get some steps in walking around the parking garage while I was receiving the day's treatment. Abigail would do the same or would take a nap. Mary and Abigail have been my strongest supporters each step of the way. They have been incredibly loving, supportive, and caring, attending to my every need.

As I pondered where to find a support group beyond my wife and daughter, I did not have to spend much time or look far. First, I received a fortuitous phone call from a fraternity brother in Tampa. He is a retired Navy JAG officer who had a successful law practice in Tampa. Unbeknownst to me, he is also a prostate cancer survivor and a current patient of Dr. Hernandez. He has been extremely supportive and upbeat during my journey, even as he was still battling leukemia and other related health issues. His frequent calls helped to put me more at ease as I prepared to undergo my cancer treatment. As we talked, it struck me that I had another support group already in place. As noted, some of my friends and colleagues from Saint Leo University, the University of South Florida (USF), as well as classmates from college and even elementary school have gone through their own journeys dealing with prostate cancer. Each had taken a different approach to deal with the disease and have shared their personal insights, which were useful.

I found another source of support in an unlikely place as I was preparing to meet with the doctors at TGH. It turned out that the dermatologist I had been going to for 30 years was retiring a couple of months after me. During my last visit to his office as a patient, he informed me that he, too, had been diagnosed with prostate cancer. We shared our thoughts about our respective diagnoses and which treatment approach to take. While I went with External Beam Radiation Therapy (EBRT), he located a urologist in Sarasota who had a good reputation for his skills in treating prostate cancer with a radical prostatectomy procedure that allowed the patient to retain urinary continence. He was able to have his surgery before the pandemic shut down local hospitals for elective procedures. As we have traveled down our individual paths on our cancer journeys, we have shared insights about our experiences in the months following our treatments. We jokingly say that our doctor-patient relationship has evolved into a "patient-patient" relationship.

I do not consider myself a deeply religious person, but after receiving my cancer diagnosis I sought support from my "higher power" to help guide me through the travails of the journey. I prayed daily and I reached out to my rabbi, Jason Rosenberg, and other friends in the local religious community. I also contacted another rabbi who is the Director of the Hillel's of the Suncoast whose daughter attended high school with my daughter. I told them of my diagnosis and they each added me to their respective weekly prayer list for a speedy recovery (Refuah Sheleima). Rabbi Rosenberg continues to check in with me periodically to make sure I am okay, both physically and spiritually. Members of our local congregation have also reached out to me to share their thoughts and good wishes. While the pandemic has kept us from seeing each other, they have helped to keep my spirits up.

Having worked at a Catholic liberal arts university for 20+ plus years, I developed wonderful caring relationships with members of the Saint Leo Abbey, the neighboring monastic community and with faculty members and staff members who are priests. One in particular, Father Michael Cooper, SJ is a member of the religion and theology faculty at Saint Leo. Father Michael came to Saint Leo in the same year I did and we both worked on the staff of the university president for some time before moving into our full-time faculty roles. He has been a wonderful, supportive friend over the past 20 years. We speak weekly and his friendship and prayers have been most beneficial. I also reached out to Abbot Isaac Comacho of the Saint Leo Abbey and Brother Lucius Amarillas, a former student who is now a monk at the Abbey studying for the priesthood. Their prayers also have helped to raise my spirits during my cancer journey. Another priest, Father Stephan Brown who grew up in Cleveland, Ohio and who had served as the Campus Minister at Saint Leo has kept me on his prayer list. Father Stephan and I have many mutual connections to our hometown of Cleveland and at times I have referred to him as my "cousin" because of our Cleveland connections. I feel certain that their support through prayers and positive thoughts have helped me along my journey.

There have been many other instances of support from friends and colleagues that have been totally surprising and very humbling. Early on in my journey and before I started radiation, two friends invited us over to their home for a Super Bowl party, which happened to be on my birthday (thank you to the NFL). They surprised me with a wonderful chocolate birthday dessert (I am one of the most die-hard chocoholics you will ever find). This helped to put me in the right frame of mind for the journey ahead. Later, upon completion of the radiation therapy in late April, I was at home one evening with Mary relaxing after dinner. Two other close friends drove over to the house for a "social distancing" post radiation therapy dessert celebration in the driveway. They brought ice cream and home-made brownies and we had a very enjoyable time together in our driveway, socially distanced to make sure we stayed safe in the midst of the pandemic. Another close friend came by regularly with protein shakes to help me maintain my weight. Also, later in the spring, a former colleague and friend from Saint Leo stopped by on his way home from work. We had a nice social distancing happy hour in the driveway, and it was very relaxing and enjoyable. I have been deeply touched by their caring gestures and their friendship.

Support has come in other, more basic forms throughout this journey. As people learned of my cancer diagnosis, they shared their thoughts and prayers in email, via text message, via phone. Some even went the "old fashioned" route of sending get well cards, often sharing thoughts about our friendship over the years. Messages have come from neighbors, elementary and high school friends, fraternity brothers, classmates from college, faculty colleagues at Saint Leo and from students who were in my classes during my time as a professor of criminal justice. These acts of support and messages have really buoyed my spirits.

In recent weeks during this journey, I have learned of other friends in Tampa and outside of Florida who have recently received a diagnosis of prostate cancer and need support, just as I did when I received my diagnosis and started my journey as a cancer patient. I have reached out to them to "pay it forward" and provide them support and friendship that has been so meaningful and helpful to me on my journey. After all, we are all in this together!

LEARNING TO ACCEPT SUPPORT

By
Bonnie Cashin Farmer

Caring for patients and their families, as broadly defined, is a core concept of the nursing profession. As a nurse I had always been much more comfortable providing care as opposed to receiving care, nurture, and support. The values inherent in being a nurse invariably extends beyond the borders of practice to my family, my role as spouse, parent, grandparent, and myself. I would rarely consider asking friends or even my family for help; for me giving support to my beloved spouse and children was easy while accepting support was infinitely more challenging.

My family has fed my soul throughout my adult life; my spouse and I began as a team of two until we eventually became a team of four with our children. We all have been there for each other, shoulder to shoulder and arm in arm in times of celebration, sorrow, and everyday life. In 2015, my immediate family had grown to include their spouses, and our four grandchildren ranging in age from four to twelve years old. Neither family lives in our immediate area yet with modern technology our family's sustained closeness fills my heart and continues to be the mainstay for my sustenance and support. My own cancer diagnosis seemed an additional burden to our families who were already devastated by their father's cancer diagnosis: so as usual I charged forward with the intent that I could handle this somewhat "minor" cancer of mine as compared to their father's cancer.

In the few weeks leading to my surgery, my spouse experienced several hospitalizations. At the time of my biopsy, I was staying overnight in my spouse's hospital room. I had to ask a close friend to drive me to my biopsy. Upon returning from the biopsy, staff provided me with ice packs. My spouse was unaware of what had transpired that day.

When meeting with the surgeon, I asked my lifelong friend from out of state to come with me to take notes and provide a third ear. Her husband stayed with my spouse who could not remain alone in our home. In true form, I naively thought that breast surgery would pose "no problem" in caring for my spouse. I would just use my "other arm" in lifting his dead weight legs. When I learned that post-op recovery included physical restrictions for both arms, I began to realize more clearly that I did have a "problem" as to how to meet his need for sustained continuity of complex care. Homecare was not involved at that time. Understandably my focus was always within the framework of caring for my spouse as opposed to dealing with my cancer.

Planning was essential to managing all the immediate details of our acute circumstances; my daughter would take me to my surgery and stay for several days. Our situation became more complicated when my spouse was readmitted to the hospital in the week before my surgery and discharged on the day of my surgery. With short notice, my brother-in- law drove three hours from out of state and covered the late day discharge. He planned to stay the next day. As my daughter and I returned home from my late day surgery, an ambulance with its lights flashing was in our driveway! In disbelief and terror, my daughter ran out of the car; her father had collapsed when unable to make the one step from the garage into the house. My brother-in-law was unable to lift him up. The next morning his brother called his spouse to come as soon as possible for additional help. They provided loving care, meals, and groceries despite a blizzard during the days it took for me to resume some balance of capability for caregiving. My spouse had no comprehension nor realization of my surgery. Today we all can even have a little chuckle that my brother-in-law had no idea what he was getting himself into when he offered to come, but at the time the seriousness of our situation was no laughing matter. Receiving assistance and support outside our immediate family, even from close friends and my spouse's brother, provided me with a gradual insight toward recognizing that trying to "do it all" would just not be sustainable on a long-term basis.

I remain eternally grateful for the support by so many given to our family during those initial turbulent times. Get well cards and wishes poured in from friends, extended family, our dentists, our work colleagues, YMCA friends, acquaintances, and even strangers from two church-based "call to care programs". Meals, homemade cornbread, and goodies filled our bodies, and our hearts as did a prayer shawl from a niece, an angel wing from another niece, and a pink hand knitted circle scarf from a friend. When we received a bouquet of flowers during one of my spouse's hospitalizations, the card read, "The girls from the pool". I slowly processed the senders' comments and began yelling, "The girls from the pool! The girls from the pool!" I momentarily forgot that I was in a hospital room. Oh, how I missed them all! The prayer shawl remains draped on a bedroom chair, the angel wing joined a cross and a lighthouse on my everyday necklace, the pink scarf much enjoyed, and a large plastic container, with every card, greeting, and loving wishes received, is easily accessible from a nearby closet.

During my surgery and initial treatments, I also received significant and meaningful support that came from both my spouse's healthcare team in addition to my own healthcare team: including personnel on the oncology unit during his hospitalizations. During one hospital discharge, the unit social worker gave us two small stone hearts which remain by our front door. My spouse and I are patients in the same multi-dimensional oncology practice located within a comprehensive outpatient facility that offers many services such as oncology radiation, varied imaging, diagnostic testing, genetic counseling, pharmacy, labs, and other specialty practices. Regardless of whether I was bringing my spouse to the "treatment room", running across the hall for my radiation treatments, or unsuccessfully disguising my tears, I genuinely felt their sensitivity, understanding, and support for the challenging duality of our circumstances. To this day I am grateful for the extreme kindness and competence of care shown to me by so many.

Early in the first year of diagnosis, I recognized the need to develop some strategies when seeing a friend or an acquaintance in the grocery store, former students, workers in local businesses and services. Crying in the grocery store while blocking an aisle just did not work for me. I created a varying set of meaningful responses which allowed me to acknowledge their support while providing me the emotional space for completing tasks like getting prescriptions, food for dinner, or just milk and eggs. I slowly became more adept with formulating responses in advance. Standing in the fresh produce aisle proved to be no place for me to share my grieving heart, acute terror for a current respiratory infection, or a litany of ongoing morbid details. Acknowledging the challenges that we were facing and thanking them for asking worked well. I could not reply that we were "fine" because we were not. My responses usually included the preface, "given our circumstances."

When reflecting upon those initial years of diagnoses and disease, my spouse has continually expressed his sorrow at his inability to support me through my own cancer. I remind him that the herculean strength in coping with the devastation of his disease was all the support that I needed. My continued support from him has been that seven years later, here he is and still doing his best every day. Our marriage had always been a source of mutual support for each other and our family; now it is just in a "different form."

As the years of living with my spouse's catastrophic disease have progressed, I also have found that constant support from friends and acquaintances changes in both form, purpose, and function. Prolonged intensive support from others outside the immediate family is not always realistic, sustainable, or necessary. I have gradually came to being more open to accepting support whenever I think it necessary or imperative as during the many continuing periods of acute medical crises. By acknowledging what I can and cannot do "given our circumstances," I have been better able to manage the challenges of caregiving combined with navigating his medical care and nurturing our quality of life together for as long as possible. My friends also have come to know that "holding steady" or "pretty good" communicates that we are okay. In our world as we live it, "holding steady" is a good thing!

My spouse and I now chuckle when people tell us how great he looks. He will often share his doubts as to "well, what would you expect them to say?" I remind him that in the first years of his disease, those same friends and acquaintances said nothing about how he looked. He knowingly smiles in a way that has always captured my heart. To my close friends I may say with a wink that "looks can be deceiving." We experience daily coping with his declining quality of life while living with incurable active cancer, forever chemotherapy treatment, and related medication side effects privately behind closed doors. The frequent friendly inquiries as to how my spouse is "doing" by friends, neighbors, and acquaintances are much appreciated. Such simple gestures of caring thoughts can communicate that they are still there and cheering us on; being there if we need them. I always express a heartfelt thank you and remain so grateful for their enduring friendships. Support surrounds us if one remains open and receptive.

I personally remind myself that oftentimes individuals mean well when, for example, they recall a "neighbor" who lived for years with a similar incurable disease. In my mind, I try not to resort to thinking that the neighbor did not know upon receiving a diagnosis with a poor prognosis for survival that they would live for another seven years! Some individuals do beat the odds and the statistics while others do not. Individuals may mean well while at the same time their comments may be off-putting. I think it is essential to remember that the intent of an individual's effort for support is really what is important. Individuals may not know what to say and can sometimes say strange things. One neighbor recently commented that recovering from her recent surgery included temporary physical restrictions which made her realize what my spouse was going through. My potentially judgmental mind could have received her comments that her physical limitations were temporary, while his were permanent. With good intentions, she was just trying to make that connection for expressing care. If one does not know what to say, I think it is perfectly acceptable and appropriate to say, "I don't know what to say." Acknowledging one's loss of words can also communicate empathy and a deeper sense of understanding.

The concept of support also provides opportunities for helping others and paying support forward. Support for others need not take time that one may not have. Support can be an attitude that communicates, "I see you and I care." Support can be in the form of an "I'm here if you need me." Although I have little extra time, I do find much satisfaction in trying to offer support in small ways. Going outside of ourselves, creating shreds of human connection despite our own circumstances, can be liberating and convey a sense of being alive; beyond just surviving. Helping others even with small gestures of kindness, praising workers in the grocery store, and vocalizing one's appreciation can make a difference. Support, however small, really is about the possibility of making a difference in one's life, including one's own life.

Support can be considered as external to self and as something one receives outside of oneself. I personally find my internal support is always there for the asking. Supporting myself in mind, body, and spirit can help to mitigate the engulfing chaos of my spouse's disease. In addition to acknowledging the positive impact of outside support, I am slowly cultivating a foundation of personal support for myself. For example, I have come to better recognize my capabilities for emotional strength and for nurturing myself as exemplified by establishing routines that I can manage. I have become much more conscious in setting boundaries for myself as to what I am willing, or not willing, to do beyond my laser focus of caregiving for my spouse. I remain a work in progress!

STRONGER TOGETHER

By
Cherie LaFlamme Genua

A topic that comes up often throughout and after treatment is support. After sharing my cancer journey on social media, I received private messages from friends or acquaintances who said things like: "My (fill in the blank) just got diagnosed with cancer… how can I help them?" Friends and family members of people with cancer often want to help, but do not know where to start. Many studies have shown that cancer patients and survivors with strong support systems tend to have a more positive outlook and better quality of life, regardless of the stage and path of treatment. Everyone who has cancer needs support—no matter how strong or independent they are. I was blessed to have a wonderful support system, all of whom took different approaches in supporting me through my journey.

Supporting a loved one with a cancer diagnosis is not a simple formula because it is not the same for everyone. Some patients on their cancer journey appreciate gifts and visits, while others prefer a text or note in their mailbox. Some have no problem reaching out for help, while others are more private. The important thing is that you attempt to show them you are thinking of them by simply trying—whatever that means to you. Send a text of encouragement or a joke to lift their spirits. Even if they do not answer, they will see it eventually and it might make them smile. Leave muffins on their doorstep with a "thinking of you card." Visit, with permission, if they are up for it. Make plans for a walk or a movie on the couch and do not be offended if and when plans are canceled at the last minute. And, remember, the challenging times continue throughout treatment and beyond. Many people will drop off a meal after the shock of the initial diagnosis (which is a kind gesture, of course), but it may come in handy further along in their treatment when the patient is fatigued or otherwise defeated. But any and every action on your part will be appreciated—even if a "thank you" note from the patient never follows. The best anyone can do is try. It goes a long way, trust me.

What did support look like for me? My husband and mother blazed the trail and were there every step of the way—on the good days, and, especially, on the bad days. My coworkers sent me flowers for every milestone, my nieces and nephews gave me stuffed animals to comfort me, and my best friend cheered me up and made me feel normal. I had the best surprise visits from out-of-town friends, meal drop-offs, and "thinking of you" cards in my mailbox from people near and far. All of this helped me remain positive and ready for each step of the journey.

My husband listened to me cry out of fear. He never once complained or made me feel like a burden. He cooked, cleaned, worked, covered me with blankets as I slept for the days following treatment, and kissed my forehead before bed. He made reservations at my favorite restaurant in the midst of chemotherapy for Valentine's Day. I remember getting dressed up, putting on my favorite chestnut-colored wig, and sitting amongst the other couples in the bustling scene. I felt normal and beautiful as we laughed the night away.

My mother set up a virtual office in the lobby of the hospital where I was receiving treatment every week. Sometimes, I would not see her all day if another chemo buddy was with me since only one person was allowed in with me at a time, but I always knew she was there. On the last day of chemo, she brought balloons and gifts. We wore matching bright lipstick and celebrated together. She was my biggest cheerleader.

My family and friends rallied around me in droves to help me get through the hard times. For starters, a different friend or family member brought me to chemo each week to keep me company over five months (highly recommended, by the way, if your cancer center allows you to have company). My chemo buddies made my chemo bag, which was filled with entertainment and goodies, relatively obsolete. We would talk about anything and everything throughout the day during treatment. They would make me laugh and I would make them laugh, too. They would comfort me during the extra challenging days when things did not seem to be going my way. My chemo buddies even took me for lunch after treatment, which was a welcomed distraction and something I looked forward to. Not the lunch itself—although I am sure the food was great, too— but rather the time spent talking and catching up.

Many people worry that they do not have the right words to say to someone dealing with cancer. But it is not what you say—it is that you are there and ready to listen. Sometimes my chemo buddies and I would talk about cancer and how I felt about it. But mostly, we would talk about our lives. I wanted to maintain some normalcy during treatment by keeping an active role in my relationships and friendships. Hearing about their kids or pets, or even asking my advice for problems at work and beyond, made me feel like I was not a cancer patient, but a friend first.

Support does not always have to be a grand gesture or an expensive gift. One of my favorite cards I received from a friend had a Helen Keller quote on the front that read: "Keep your face to the sunshine and you cannot see the shadows. It is what the sunflowers do." The card was beautifully illustrated, but the message penetrated my soul on a day when I needed it most. It encouraged me to seek out the happy aspects of each day and focus on the positives of my life. For instance, I was doing well as I progressed through treatment, I had health insurance, I had friends and family who cared greatly for me. By focusing on the good in life, it helps to banish the negative thoughts and feelings that creep into our minds. The "why me?" questions that drag us down. This hand-selected card still sits in my kitchen and reminds me every day to make the best of any situation. And it should remind you that a card, text, or note can go a long way in making someone's day or week.

Cancer can be lonely. Spend time with your friend—you can make them feel like they once did before cancer became a major part of their life. My best friend was amazing at this. She was there for the "cancer" things, yes. She helped bandage me after my surgery and dropped off food and supplies. But she got me out of the house and gave me things to look forward to. We did a "paint night" for my birthday while sipping wine and laughing at our lack of artistic ability. We even went on an international trip together towards the end of immunotherapy to celebrate our friendship. We went on walks around the neighborhood often. Suggest a walk with your friend, too. The change of scenery, fresh air, and conversation will do wonders for their mental state.

I was lucky enough to have others in my community who had unfortunately gone through their own cancer journeys. My husband's good friend and college roommate is a Ewing's Sarcoma Cancer survivor. He and his wife offered tons of indispensable advice throughout my own journey. His positivity and "charge ahead" attitude helped me crawl out of some dark places. He is thriving and I admire his strength. I met some wonderful women in my age group who had similar breast cancer stories, as well. We talked about anything and everything—from hair loss to having children to radiation burns and beyond. Having people in your circle who know what you are feeling helps. Even if you do not personally know anyone with a cancer diagnosis, there are support groups everywhere with people willing to lend an ear or offer help. I joined a twelve-week exercise and wellness program through my gym and met a wonderful group of people. Ask your oncologist for more information on local groups. A simple Google online search will also return many results, as well. Or contact me—I am always willing to listen.

Support also came from within, too. Not just through self-care measures, such as relaxing baths, face masks, cozy socks, and heated blankets; but also, from being aware of my own needs and knowing when I needed a break. At work, if I did not feel well, I would not try to work through the pain or exhaustion. I would go home for the day and pick back up after I had time to rest, or I would rest in a quiet spare office. At home, I knew better than trying to clean my whole house and hired people to help me with that effort.

I would accept meals from friends or family members who offered—not just for me, but for my spouse who took on the bulk of the household chores and meal-planning. I put myself out there and shared my story on social media, not for sympathy but to educate and help others who may be dealing with a similar story. Or, perhaps to inspire young women like me to perform self-breast exams and get to know their bodies in case anything ever feels "off." I received private messages from high school classmates and women with whom I have studied abroad in college stating they are now diligent about performing monthly breast exams because of my social media posts. Plus, comments of strength and prayers from others who you may not have talked to in a while help to keep you going, too. Speaking of social media, it is a great place to find a support system and community. For instance, searching by hashtags such as #breastcancer or #ovariancancer or #cancerthriver will help you find other people dealing with a similar diagnosis. Many in this community welcome and encourage messages from others with questions or advice. It is a great way to not feel so alone throughout your journey. People share the good, the bad, and the ugly parts of their cancer journeys, and their posts might answer the very question on your mind at that moment. I was inspired by women sharing mastectomy photos or pictures of their bald, beautiful heads. I highly recommend using Facebook and Instagram to connect you to other wonderful people fighting battles alongside you—you never know who you will meet that will inspire you or vice versa!

Through social media, I also found non-profit organizations with various missions that were helpful along my journey. For instance, I found a local non-profit that delivered power lift reclining chairs to help women after breast surgery. Who knew that type of service existed? My mother found another organization who sent mini colorful boxing gloves to encourage women to "fight pretty" (fightingpretty.org). I received soft knit caps, wig support, and even free home cleaning services during active treatment. Some non-profits help pay bills if you are out of work by providing grants and there are others that send gift cards for food or groceries. There are countless resources out there—all you have to do is find them (or ask someone else to help you find them!).

All in all, support comes from a myriad of places in a variety of ways. Yes, it will come from your partner, family members, and friends. It will also come from support groups or social media channels. It will come from strangers turned friends in your community. You can receive support through non-profits organizations. Support can, and should, come from within too. It will come in the form of texts, calls, social media posts, cards, and emails. It might come from gifts or flowers that remind you that people are cheering you on every day. Remember, support is personal. There is no wrong or right answer on how to best support your loved one with cancer. Support means trying—by whatever feels comfortable to you or your cancer patient in need.

ACCEPTING SUPPORT

BY
Burt Harres

It is difficult for me to imagine how anyone who is diagnosed with cancer would not want to seek and accept support. The journey of a cancer patient can be emotionally and physically draining. Then again, each individual will eventually determine to what degree, if any, he or she will seek and accept the support of others. In my case, from the day of my initial diagnosis through the present day, I openly sought and accepted support. However, I believe my support would be considered "narrow and deep" as opposed to "wide and shallow."

Although I led a very public life as a college administrator, I am basically a private person. I have a few remarkably close friends and many acquaintances. I like to keep my personal business just that way…personal. So, I decided to keep my support group to a relatively small number with friends and colleagues who either needed to know my condition and/or whose love and guidance I valued. That is why I describe my support group as narrow in number but deep with their compassion, most notably my fiance, Marilyn, and sons, Michael and David.

Conversely, I did not see any benefit in telling everyone I knew or posting on social media that I was diagnosed with prostate cancer. I personally found it to be very emotionally and physically draining when I informed my family, closest friends and select colleagues about my condition. I determined that I wanted to spend my emotional and physical energy on the battle ahead of me instead of sharing my diagnosis with many people. I subscribed to the proverbial expression that "less is more."

Please do not misconstrue the term "shallow" as meaning inconsequential. The friends, acquaintances, and colleagues who I never told and never knew about my condition are wonderful people. It is just that, in my opinion, most folks are living busy lives with their own triumphs, trials, and tribulations. When they ask, "how are you doing," they do not expect a "sincere" answer. That does not mean it is a bad thing. It is just that responding "pretty good" is just a common practice for small talk and discussing cancer is definitely not small talk.

The noted author, Eckhart Tolle, asserts, "When you complain, you make yourself a victim. Leave the situation, change the situation, or accept it. All else is madness." I know that once I accepted my prostate cancer diagnosis, I resolved to not consider myself to be a "victim." From that point forward, it was significantly easier for me to embrace the support I needed. I will be forever grateful for the support that I accepted and continue to receive on my journey as a cancer patient. I consider myself to be a religious person. I am a Roman Catholic and I believe in the power of prayer. For me, my prayers to God provided me with tremendous spiritual support. I will be forever grateful for the support I received from my then fiancé, my sons, and my uncles and aunts. I also confided in several of my closest male friends. Since I had to leave work early to receive cancer treatments, my professional colleagues were extremely supportive during my absences from work.

I would be remiss if I did not mention the many anonymous prostate cancer patients whom I met in the waiting area of my oncologist's office. Unlike many stark and cold waiting areas that are commonplace in most doctors' offices, I often referred to the design as resembling a "men's clubhouse." There are two large areas with cushy leather couches and chairs in a rectangular layout that encourage patients to interact with each other. The patients were almost always at different stages in their treatment plans. The conversations I had enabled me to ask questions to men who were farther along in their treatment plan and to offer encouragement and answer questions to others whose treatment plan was not as advanced as mine. I am convinced that these numerous conversations among men battling the same cancer provided an incredible amount of mutual support to us all.

At this point in my journey as a cancer patient, I offer the following lessons learned:

- People living with cancer often benefit from the practical help and advice they receive from others who have lived through similar situations. Support groups bring people together. They provide a safe forum for exchanging perspectives, sharing concerns, and gaining confidence to face the future. If misery loves to enlarge itself with more misery, surely heartfelt friendship and kinship enlarges itself with more heartfelt friendship and kinship. Be open to accepting and nurturing healthy, faithful friendships and kinships. Accepting support can make a positive difference in one's cancer journey.

CHAPTER THREE:

HOPE

HOPE AND THE PATIENT WITH CANCER

By
Richard E. Farmer

Hope is indeed a complex issue for all human beings to deal with. While this complexity applies to all human beings, it is particularly relevant to those whose illness or age is such that it is likely to be more imperative. Hope provides a livable statement about quality of life. As an alternative to the idea of hope as a pathway for disease-fighting, hope can provide a set of statements or directions to be followed for the living of a quality life. While the concrete approach determining a sort of mechanistic attitude is a normal human process, hope can be useful for conceptualizing a much broader approach to living. The dimensions of this are endless and usually involve other people, family, friends and perhaps even volunteering yourself to assist others in need.

There are many ways of examining the concept of hope as it applies to the cancer patient. At its very core, hope and the patient may be seen through the lens of the quality of life or lifestyle, a religious orientation and faith, and the belief in the human soul.

As an individual diagnosed more than 7 years ago with Multiple Myeloma cancer and having served as a volunteer moderator for a support group, I have been struck by the reliance on the part of some cancer patients who place significant emphasis on clinical trials and research, and the desire to "battle and fight" the disease in order to seek cure and avoid untimely death. This emphasis also applies to healthcare providers and researchers, many of whom are the very originators of this focus. Offering hope supports that singular human need to achieve another state of being. As a need, hope is more than an emotional state with something that could be different in our lives.

Hope is a multifaceted human need that drives one to achieve or craft one's life in a certain direction. More than a guide or roadmap for ourselves, our families, our friends and beyond, hope can influence the essence of every fundamental human behavior from birth to death.

Hope can produce a quality of life which may be considered a lifestyle. That is, our daily behavior from birth onwards is built around a series of ideas, principles, concepts, and other's thoughts that form a belief system and ultimately organized as a lifestyle. While the concept of lifestyle is a complicated phenomenon, the idea of grouping the many forms of individual human behavior into a set of mostly observable behaviors can have at its core, the idea of hope. Hope may well be the driving force as we traverse our way through life. And part of this is the idea that hope is an amazing gift from God which underlies the very essence of a positive quality of life or standard by which we live from birth to death.

In many organized religions, hope is part of the foundation of religious faith which is built around the omnipresent force commonly referred to as the concept of God. And, as some religions have espoused, the human soul is the person's window to God, which guides our thoughts and beliefs about our future, and ultimately to our understanding about the hereafter. Hope also helps to form three other aspects of human behavior.

These three beliefs are the belief in the human soul, belief in our own future, and finally, a belief in the hereafter. Aside from biological growth and development, the human being also learns, accepts, and inculcates into our being the beliefs in the human soul, our own future, and the hereafter forming our human core. Hope, then, becomes a primary vehicle for understanding human existence.

So, how do we make sense out of this? As mentioned, my own interest in this topic grew out of my volunteer work as a moderator for a virtual support group for people with various forms of blood cancer. In this work, I quickly noted the almost exclusive interest on the part of participants in medications they were taking, clinical trials they were participating in, details about their chemotherapy designs, and related topics.

Initially, I was shocked to listen to the conversation. As a psychologist, I had much more anticipated discussion questions about, "What are you feeling? How are you coping? What is your family doing to help you? Are you ever angry about getting cancer? If so, how do you express yourself?" And to my professional amazement, these discussion points never came up and when asked if they were interested in talking about this, there was only some quiet grumbling.

The good news is that silence almost always works, so after a moment or two, one brave soul said, "You know, I always wanted to know what it will feel like when the "end" for me is near." Understandably, this generated a good deal of healthy discussion. So, from a hope perspective perhaps what I call Medication Talk is really Help Talk organized in a way that is emotionally acceptable to the participants.

As mentioned earlier, hope can also be viewed as a form of quality of life or lifestyle in which some have built their style of living around the concept. Virtually everything they do involves some consideration of hope. One's personal thinking about self, spouses, extended and close-in family, siblings, employers, friends and acquaintances, neighbors and virtually all others that we have contact with have hope woven into those relationships. Hope that it will remain the same, or that it will change for the better, or somehow be different. Hope is tightly woven into our very essence or being and is the principle upon which we judge and evaluate virtually all our thinking concerning the past, the present, and the future.

From a practical point of view, the concept of hope is difficult to understand, especially in the presence of catastrophic disease. Disease challenges us to live beyond the confines of the disease as we know it or come to understand it. One way of understanding this is to examine the emotional role of medications at the center of disease treatment, especially cancer treatment. The principal advocates of this are first the practitioner who provides the diagnostic understanding of the disease and prescribes the medication to "fight" the disease.

Second are the patients who often develop a fixation around the current medication, the clinical research around new medications, and the overall effectiveness of both. What is interesting to note is this author's own experience with his multiple oncology physicians wherein the regular monthly appointments are almost completely focused on the efficacy of the medications that fight the symptoms of the disease itself and the side-effects of the disease fighting medications. Only under a few rare circumstances have we had a conversation about feelings, emotional coping strategies, and end-of-life expectations.

Hope does not equal living per se. Some have the idea that if they go through life embracing hope that they are truly living. Yet, hope alone does not and could not define living. If all our ideas, actions, behaviors, thoughts, and the like are based solely on hope, then indeed we are deferring the present reality for the future which is, by definition, hope oriented. While living, meaning the past, present, and future, does contain elements of hope, it is the totality of the hope concept that is problematic as it could keep us from what is happening because we are focused only on hope elements for the future. It is a sort of childhood version of, "when I grow up, I'm going to be...." Hope for the past, present, and future is necessary, but it is the totality of it that does not constitute living in and of itself.

As mentioned, hope feeds the soul with a sense of identity which enables the person to live beyond the current situation that individuals find themselves in. As humans, we are complex individuals who are relatively close, but not a copy of one another. We are created with the idea of a soul or a sense of self that combines our past, present, and the future. This is best understood as a combination of behaviors, religious beliefs, thoughts, feelings, guidelines, cultural belief systems and the like that can structure how we think and behave. This is most especially the case as we contemplate future thoughts, wishes, desires, and behaviors. How our soul is developed will determine in part how we will behave in the future. And for many, our souls have an exceptionally large religious or spiritual component which serves to help guide us through all our days on Earth.

This is especially the case for those of us with a terminal illness whose end can and is predicted in terms of time-based sequences and levels of disease. The longer the time with the disease and its level provides a statistical determination of the average life span. Hence, the role of hope and its foundation in God becomes even more important to the cancer patient as one prepares for life hereafter. Perhaps the final and most significant statement about hope is the question about God being eternal life. As cancer patients and others face the probability of near death, the idea that God is about eternal life gathers increasing importance and meaning. As human beings facing imminent death, the idea of the hereafter takes on ever-increasing importance. And, for those of us raised with a concept of God as part of our intellect and being, at the very essence of hope there is an ever-strong belief that God is responsible for our hopeful belief in our daily existence and in the afterlife.

Even though cancer patients must follow a structured path of treatment for disease resolution, that path does not preclude additional elements which have a broader appeal and usefulness for the patient. In fact, an attitude of belief that the future may be pre-determined because of the disease, adding other dimensions like hope to one's living can strengthen one's approach and add richness to their quality of living.

To this end then, hope is a gift and becomes the essence of a quality-of-life issue for us. We surround ourselves with the idea that hope is a gift, and one which has been nurtured by ourselves over time and often nurtured by other people in our lives. We have been taught or otherwise learned that the idea of hope provides one of the principal ways to achieve happiness in life even within the context of catastrophic disease. As we move through our own individual stages of development, hope is a human quality that enables us to create opportunities for positivity and peace of heart.

MY HOPE

By
David W. Persky

What is hope?

According to Merriam Webster Collegiate Dictionary (10th Ed.) hope is "desire accompanied by expectation of or belief in fulfillment. expectation of fulfillment or success; something hoped for."

Over the course of my cancer journey, hope has been ever present in my thoughts as I dealt with prostate cancer. When the initial PSA result came back from the Cleveland Clinic, I fervently hoped that an error was made in the test and that the PSA was not as high as indicated, or perhaps a lab technician had misread the results. When the original result was confirmed with the second PSA test at TGH, I continued to hope that an error was made, and that the PSA was not really as high as previously indicated. My hope was partially realized because the second PSA number was lower, but still too high.

As my physician conducted the biopsy and analyzed the results of the MRI, bone scan and CT scan, I hoped that the diagnosis was incorrect. Perhaps it was just a case of External Benign Prostatic Hyperplasia (EBPH), or enlargement of the prostate. EBPH is a relatively common condition in men over the age of 40 and its frequency increases as men age. Forty years ago, the common treatment for EBPH was surgery, but now it can be treated with medication.

As an eternal optimist, when the biopsy came back positive for cancer, I shifted my hope to have the cancer localized in the prostate and to have the cancer removed as soon as feasibly possible. I prepared myself that the cancer would be removed, and I hoped that I would not have to undergo chemotherapy as part of the treatment. My hope was realized and the bone scan and CT scan each came back clear indicating that the cancer was localized and had not metastasized outside of the prostate. I was feeling surprisingly good, yet I was a bit apprehensive as to what was going to follow.

I started the radiation therapy hoping that the EBRT would kill the cancer and that there would be no negative residual side effects. The treatments were painless, and I completed the twenty-five sessions with no complications that I knew of. I had no difficulty in urination or with bowel movements. (I think the doctors were a bit surprised). One day as I was getting out of the shower, my wife saw some radiation spots on my buttocks and not knowing what they were, we were both concerned. The spots did not itch and were not painful. I had a dermatologist check them out and there was no cause for concern. It may have been radiation dermatitis, but it was nothing to worry about and the spots had faded over time in the subsequent weeks and months. Subsequent PSA tests revealed the cancer was "undetectable" as the PSA scores were under 0.1; wonderful news! Although I was in remission, the physicians decided to continue the treatment – Androgen Deprivation Therapy (ADT) to ensure the cancer would not return. Now into 10 months of my journey, I have shifted my hope: I now hope to end hormone therapy to avoid further night sweats, frequent trips to the bathroom at night and the other possible side effects from the therapy. I would like to be able to return to a reasonable fitness program to help regain muscle mass that has deteriorated from the ADT. I want to get rid of my "stick" arms and legs! I want to have a good quality of life so I can fully enjoy whatever time I may have remaining.

I have a more overriding universal hope in regard to cancer. I hope that research initiatives around the nation and the world will find a cure for prostate cancer and all other forms of cancer. We are in the middle of the worst pandemic since the Spanish Flu of 1918 and millions of people worldwide have suffered from this brutal virus. On a personal level, I hope to avoid infection from the COVID-19 virus and that the vaccines recently developed in the United States and elsewhere are successful in defeating the virus.

HOPE AND A PEACEFUL HEART

By
Bonnie Cashin Farmer

Within three plus months after my spouse's diagnosis, he lost fifty per cent of his vertebral height: meaning the cancer caused his spine to collapse and thus severely altered his spinal structure, respiratory function, and other essential esophageal and gastrointestinal functions. He remained acutely ill for an extended period. His impaired ability to swallow resulted in food becoming stuck in his throat and subsequent regurgitation. During a hospitalization for aspiration pneumonia, he underwent an esophageal dilation procedure with general anesthesia to address the narrowing of his esophagus. My adult children and I waited in a room adjacent to where the procedure was taking place.

After some period of waiting, the physician for this procedure approached us in a hurried manner and requested that I come with him immediately. A respiratory code had been called; my spouse was not coming out of the anesthesia! As I entered the procedure room, he was flailing his arms, gasping for breath, and struggling with the anesthesiologist and staff trying to administer oxygen to him. Within seconds the room was filled with hospital staff responding to the code. All of us were screaming, "Breathe, Breathe, Breathe!" I knew not one individual in this crowded room of medical strangers. I frantically asked anyone who could, "please call the hospitalist for the oncology floor and ask him to come immediately!"

The hospitalist had been present throughout his prior and present admissions. He was there in a matter of minutes. His presence provided the most appreciated support to my children and me. Our daughter and son were brought in shortly after. My beloved spouse of forty-five years was deteriorating rapidly. The hospitalist told me that he most likely would not survive more than three hours at most – no time to call his brothers two hours away, no time to say a final goodbye, no time left at all. This was "it". Yes, intubation was offered and yes, to my dismay, I briefly considered it. As a nurse I know that intubation for someone in my spouse's fragile condition was a slippery slope at best. My feet were being held to the fire.

My mind and my heart raced with thoughts of intubation and the possibility of just one more day, one more hour, yet I knew without any doubt that my spouse would not want that. The anesthesiologist then offered sedation for him and wanted me to be aware that such a medication could hasten his death. If there was anything that I could do so that my beloved spouse of forty-five years would not die in this horrific and tortuous manner, then I would be strong enough to do it. I turned to the anesthesiologist and said in a clear and unwavering voice, "give it to him." Because the physicians thought that he might die en route to the ICU, our children, myself, and staff, all went on the service elevator with my spouse on the stretcher. We were literally running down the long corridors of the hospital. Once in the ICU, the children and I were asked to wait outside. I refused in quite a loud manner, my spouse was dying and I was not going to leave him. We then agreed to wait inside the ICU by the exit door where we had a direct view of my dying spouse's room. The two-panel glass door to his ICU room was of the kind that open automatically from the center. Upon closing the doors, staff then very quickly transferred him from the stretcher to the ICU bed and, within a matter of seconds, re-opened them for us to enter.

As the doors opened, all three of us saw my spouse, the father of our beautiful children, sitting quietly up in the bed, and looking around as if to say, "what is the big fuss?" We were completely speechless. The ICU physician urgently entered the room, all while quickly looking back and forth between his notes and my spouse, and said, "oh, I must be in the wrong room – my apologies." As he turned to leave, I replied that he was not in the wrong room. The ICU physician glanced several times at my spouse as if carefully studying him. "But I just received his report of being in an acute crisis!" He said that he would be right back. Still speechless, the three of us stood there and wondered out loud what had happened here. The three of us were in real shock while my spouse was calm, gasping no more, and had no memory or understanding of the circumstances. Soon he was discharged from the ICU and returned to his room on the oncology floor. The hospital staff graciously allowed both my daughter and I to stay through that night.

Throughout the next day there was a steady stream of staff stopping by the room. Oncology staff came in to say that they had "heard" that he had quite an "event" down in the procedure room. The anesthesiologist, the esophageal physician, staff from the respiratory code, the hospital social worker, and several others came to check on him and say "hello" as if they wanted to see him with their own eyes. He was discharged home several days later. The hospitalist told us he was preparing to leave for the day when he received the early evening call from the procedure room: his computer was turned off and his coat was in his hands as he began walking out his office door. A few years later and a change of his position, he became and remains our palliative care physician. My spouse and I like to frequently remind him of his prominence within our family tapestry. He knows and we know, something beyond ourselves, beyond medicine, and certainly beyond understanding or explanation happened on that unforgettable day. Although the word "miracle" was never uttered that day, my children, myself, and others recognized and experienced a force much greater than ourselves: for me, it was Divine Intervention.

Several weeks later I found myself in a funk with none of my usual attempts of tricking myself into thinking I was okay working. I ultimately ended up prostrating myself on the kitchen floor and wailed uncontrollably until there was no more. Once again in my lifetime, I turned myself completely over to the omnipresent power that has always been present within me and by my side. Such a spiritual presence nurtures a peaceful and grateful heart in my resolve to care for my spouse to the absolute best of my abilities: it is good, it is enough, it sustains me.

I have always been a spiritual and inquiring individual seeking understanding of the world around me. Although my entire childhood was deeply rooted within a Christian orientation, many decades ago I chose not to seek affirmation of my faith within any one organized religion. I have come to recognize and respect the many worldwide ways one might express their understanding of an omnipresent presence of a God or not that guides and informs how one lives. For many, faith may be an external force of formal or informal doctrine. I have long regarded that the primacy of faith comes from within. We all have potential to call up our own faith, our own strength, and support ourselves while recognizing that we are human.

Hope is often considered as a positive aspiration, yet hope can also be an impediment as evidenced in false hope. False hope can diminish opportunities for meaningful growth of self and others. Sometimes we do not know what to hope for and sometimes we do.

Hope speaks to being multidimensional in nature. The very presence of hope in one's life can shape how persons see and experience the world around them. The intent of Hope can also shift in meaning and one's expression of hope. Hope can go beyond what you hope for as evidenced by my spouse's outcome on that day in the ICU. I had not even hoped for such an outcome yet my hope and steadfast commitment toward a "good death" for him underscored much of my decision-making. My own expressions of hope continue to be varied and range from both day to day living or worse moment to moment living in an acute crisis to thinking of how I see the remainder of my life unfolding in the presence of cancer and disease. Despite these ever-changing challenges, I remain grateful for the presence of hope to sustain me and provide confidence for the continued sustenance to my soul.

WOODEN DOLLHOUSE

By
Cherie LaFlamme Genua

When I was eight years old, I hoped for a specific dollhouse as a Christmas gift from Santa Claus. I saw it on a television advertisement, and I could not get it out of my head. It was large, wooden, and filled with doll-sized furniture in pastel hues. It even had patterned wallpaper in the bathroom. I loved the thought of having a little playground for my dolls where I could let my imagination run wild. I hoped for it and it showed up, like magic, on Christmas morning. Likewise, when I was sixteen, I hoped for a cherry red sports car. That hope did not materialize but I did get a sensible automobile to drive to and from school. And, when I went on my very last "first date," I hoped that man would one day be my husband (he ended up being more than what I hoped for). My hopes and wishes over the years made me realize that as humans, we hope for a lot. It is the reason we stop at the convenience store on the way home from work to grab a lottery ticket. When you are poor, there is nothing to hope for more than some extra money to pay the bills. The first time our foot hits the pavement on a lackluster jog, we hope we would one day be able to run a marathon (well, that is wishful thinking, for me anyway).

And when we are sick, we hope for health.

For cancer patients, the future is often unknown. But it is hope that keeps us going to get through treatments and the hardships that come along with a cancer diagnosis. Hope is the belief that a positive outcome lies ahead, even if it feels nebulous. Hope can also be fleeting and fragile, especially when things do not seem to be going our way. If we start to lose hope—in ourselves, in our medical team, in the support from our family and friends—it can be detrimental to our psyche and our well-being as we navigate the unknown of being a cancer patient.

When I was diagnosed with breast cancer at the age of 34, I hoped to be cured and find my way into remission as soon as humanly possible. I had things to do. I had personal and professional goals to crush. I had trips to

Italy and Machu Picchu that were calling my name. I was ready to start a family. I wanted to look in the rearview mirror and have cancer disappear further behind me as I drove away and headed back towards my normal life. Now, of course, we all know that it is not that simple. A cancer diagnosis is never truly in the rearview mirror, but when I began my cancer journey, I based everything on the hope that it would. But as much as I hoped my cancer journey would soon be a distant memory, I mostly used hope to get me through the darkness. It catapulted me forward towards brighter days that I hoped would come my way.

I found hope to be a driving factor in how I got through my own cancer journey. It is still a belief I cling on to and it always will be. But It was not always easy to hang on to hope while staring cancer in the eye. There were days that felt hopeless. With vivid memory, I recall catching a glimpse of my reflection in the water-stained mirror of the chemo room bathroom during my fourteenth treatment. My face was bright pink and blotchy; my body was puffy. My fingers swelled up like balloons to the point where I could not wear my wedding rings. My head was bald and uncovered. To say I looked bad was an understatement. Even though I only had two chemotherapy infusions left, at that moment, I did not think I would make it through to the finish line. The hope deep inside that drove me forward through the first thirteen treatments was missing in the fluorescent lighting of the stark tiled bathroom that day. I was void of hope and I found the dark thoughts creeping their way back in. The emotions I was feeling were defeating. But I knew I had to splash water on my face and summon the hope needed to fight another day, week, and month so I could ring that bell on the final day of chemotherapy. Getting there would inch me towards the next hope of clear scans at the conclusion of treatment. My days of hoping for a doll house were gone—hope these days looked more like pink ribbons and a cure.

So, how did I get there? How did I manifest hope and forge ahead?

A lot of my hope came from my oncology team and from the advancements that have been made in breast cancer research. I felt hopeful in the plan and strategy that my team of doctors laid out for me. Every time I saw my oncologist, he reassured me that I was doing well with my treatments. He reviewed my bloodwork before each chemotherapy infusion and allowed me to advance forward. He felt my tumor decrease in size over time. And he read my pathology results that showed no evidence of disease after surgery. My belief in hope was restored, giving me the boost needed to carry on and continue towards my next phase of treatment, which was radiation.

But even though the science behind my diagnosis helped me understand more about my treatment plan and my side effects, there was no science or strategy behind the idea of hope. I could not read medical journals or textbooks about how to hope. Hope had to come from deep within. I could not flip on a switch towards hope and healing, but I could lean into ideas and activities that helped hope to emerge. Things like communicating with other survivors—more on this in a minute—and doing activities that made me happy and kept me positive…those kinds of things kept me hopeful. Also, hope is not a linear process—it ebbs and flows depending on the day—but being able to recognize and accept that made hope feel attainable.

Hope came in the form of sharing my journey and talking to others to hear theirs. I met a wonderful group of women who all, unfortunately, shared the fact that we were diagnosed with breast cancer. I met them through support groups and organically through everyday life. When I went for an eye exam and was asked my medical history, the woman doing my check-up told me that she was a survivor, too. This happened often—it is almost as if we all had the scarlet letter "C" branded on us, only visible to other survivors. "I'm a 15-year survivor," I can recall one woman saying to me with a wink. It was this version of hope—others like me who were alive and thriving—that got me through many difficult days.

A woman I follow on social media who was also fighting breast cancer in her 30s shared the following quote, "What Cancer Cannot Do: Cancer is so limited. It cannot cripple LOVE. It cannot shatter HOPE. It cannot corrode FAITH. It cannot destroy PEACE. It cannot kill FRIENDSHIP. It cannot suppress MEMORIES. It cannot silence COURAGE. It cannot invade the SOUL. It cannot steal eternal LIFE. It cannot conquer the SPIRIT."

I added that quote to the background of my phone and internalized this quote so much that it became part of me. Those beautiful words felt so empowering as I navigated the dark and unknown world of cancer. And those words were all true: cancer can and will do a lot of horrible things to us and our bodies and mental states, but it could not stop me from loving and hoping. Not if I did not let it, of course.

But as hopeful stories of women surviving breast cancer and getting further into remission inspired me, stories of recurrence or death often sent me into a spiral. I wondered how these women and men remained hopeful when receiving less-than-encouraging news from their oncology teams. When told that one's cancer has returned or they have limited time left on this earth, hope might be the last thing on their mind. Fear, sadness, anger—those are some emotions that come to mind, whereas hope might get shattered along the way. A serious illness, like cancer, is a reminder that life is not infinite. Yet, it is on the darkest days when hope becomes the most powerful belief we have.

I felt similarly when meeting with my oncology team about my "survivorship care plan." This meeting indicated a transition from treatment to post-treatment living. For me, it symbolized a return to normal life; that is, a time when my weekly schedule is no longer dictated by chemotherapy, radiation, blood work, immunotherapy, and other appointments. Survivorship is a graduation, so to speak. In the meeting, we talked about lingering side effects and the ways my body and mind changed. We also discussed what recurrence looks like and the signs and symptoms to look out for. Later on, that night—my mind still spinning from the survivorship meeting—I sat at my kitchen table and flipped through pages and pages of topics. I read about the ways in which the kind of chemotherapy I received could lead to long-term heart damage, or how weight gain was an unfortunate side effect many breast cancer survivors faced. I learned that the mental fogginess I was experiencing could stay with me for years after treatment and how strength training is critical, since the medication I am on could cause damage to my bone health. I read about relationships, sexual health, and mental health.

Although I knew many of these lasting and lingering side effects, seeing them listed in a fifty-page packet was overwhelming. I remember feeling my hope fraying as I flipped through the pages. Aside from being hopeful that I would stay in remission, I also had to hope that I would not experience many of the possible side effects in the future. I had to hope that my heart would stay healthy and that eating the occasional piece of cake would not send my body into a downward spiral towards cancer recurrence. I had to hope that my hip pain I was experiencing was arthritis and not bone cancer. I had to hope that this laundry list of worries and fears would soon live in the back of my mind as I attempted to live and enjoy my life.

I took a last sip of tea, took off my glasses, and closed my pink survivorship care plan folder. My hope came back into focus. I smiled to myself as I realized how grateful I was to have an oncology team so invested in my health and well-being. Hope is often crippled by fear, loneliness, and a slew of emotions, but it is also there to remind you that you are not alone as you navigate a scary time in your life. There are always people in your corner putting together pink packets, thinking of you, and sending positivity your way. And there is always the hope that you will get your very own wooden dollhouse filled with love, memories, courage, and support that will keep you moving forward, even when you are not sure you can get through another day.

THE GIFT OF HOPE

By
Burt Harres

"Hope" has many definitions as evidenced in The Oxford Dictionary. One definition that was helpful in my journey as a cancer patient is attributed to the American author and screenwriter, Ray Bradbury. Bradbury stated, "Action is hope. There is no hope without action." I believe it is important to differentiate between "hope" and "wishful thinking." Cancer patients who are hopeful are actively trying to investigate and implement the best path of action while taking into consideration the obstacles. Wishful thinking is passively going through the motions as if in a state of denial about actual circumstances.

Duane Bidwell Ph.D. and Donald Batisky M.D. analyzed vast amounts of data from a diverse group of children suffering from end-stage renal failure. These researchers identified five main pathways to hope applicable to everyone:

- Maintaining identity by continuing to participate in activities and relationships that help patients retain a sense of self outside diagnosis and treatment. It is important to recognize and embrace the idea that you are much more than a cancer diagnosis. To the extent that you are physically able, continuing to embrace prior activities including work, family, and recreational activities is particularly important.
- Realizing community through formal and informal connections that help patients understand that they are not alone in living with disease. This community is made real through conversation, visitation, consultation, and participation in daily activities. As appropriate, continuing to maintain current relationships and even develop new ones will reinforce to you that you are a multi-faceted individual, and not just somebody with a disease.
- Claiming control by taking an active role in treatment by setting goals, self-advocating, monitoring, and maintaining one's own health. By continuing to remember that you are the center of your treatment will help you to feel much more connected with the

process. As the patient, you must remember that you are in charge of what is done to and with you. Understanding the specific details of what is or will be happening removes surprises and allows you to better accept what is happening to and with your body.
- Tending to spirituality, activated through religious, spiritual, and other contemplative practices. Consider developing a spiritual and/or religious interest and/or commitment. Understanding that our lives will continue albeit in a different form throughout time. And, joining with others in the practice of our spirituality provides us with the opportunity to enjoy a colleagueship with others and thus reduce the sense of loneliness that we can possibly experience strictly by ourselves.
- Developing wisdom, which involves gaining pragmatic, medical wisdom derived from one's own experience and finding ways to "give back." Wisdom is a practical entity that demonstrates not only what we have learned about our health situation but also provides us with an opportunity to tell others. In this sense, teaching is an important or even critical element to the process of both learning about and expressing our hope.

These authors conclude, "the pathways are not hierarchical in any way, you can access hope through any of these pathways and all of them. The more of them you can access, the better." In my journey as a cancer patient, I know that, at one point or another, I entered each of the pathways to hope identified by Bidwell and Batisky and offer the following thoughts as these pathways relate to me:

There is a thin line between hope and wishful thinking. That line is an unwavering commitment to truth and reality. Wishful thinking encourages passivity and fosters denial, whereas hope represents action injected with positivity.

When diagnosed with cancer, maintaining a positive attitude can be difficult. Cancer patients confront a variety of obstacles and hurdles, including the side effects of the illness and treatment as well as feelings of fear, anger, depression, and loneliness. For patients with cancer, hope is what enables them to endure treatments as well as social and personal adversities.

A cancer patient's family, doctors, nurses, social workers, friends, colleagues, and clergy, among others, can play a significant role in creating and activating pathways of hope for a cancer patient. This means that these individuals can be and are great sources of hope.

The impact that hope can have on a cancer patient's recovery process is strongly supported both through empirical research and theoretical approaches as evidenced by the work of Ernest Rosenbaum M.D. and David Spiegel M.D. of Stanford University. Rosenbaum and Spiegel asserted that, "Health professionals believe that a combination of medical therapy, adoption of healthy lifestyles, medical prevention, and supportive care offers the best chance to maintain a patient's quality of life. Such comprehensive care addresses a wide range of needs, from relieving the physical symptoms of cancer and cancer therapy to satisfying the craving for intellectual, creative, and spiritual sustenance. Satisfaction of these diverse needs demonstrates the powerful connection between mind and body. Obtaining relief from pain, nausea, or fatigue, for example, restores a sense of calm. Sufficient sleep, appropriate exercise, and good nutrition are energizing. Discussing one's negative feelings candidly with others can diminish their effect. Learning to control blood pressure and heart rate through such means as biofeedback and self-hypnosis can foster a sense of personal power. Exploring one's creative potential can lead to joy and transcendence."

From a personal perspective, I am a Christian and a Roman Catholic. As a Christian, I believe that faith, hope, and love are theological virtues, gifts from God to help us in our journey on earth and eventually in heaven. The beliefs of the Catholic Church inform us that hope, as a virtue, lies in a mean between the extremes of two vices: presumption and despair. In a perfect world, there would be no suffering. Unfortunately, for many cancer patients, physical and mental suffering become part of life. The words "hope' and "suffering" do not seem to belong in the same sentence. But hope is exactly what is needed to stay engaged in living while shouldering the burden of an uncertain future. The opposite of hope is "despair", and despair can be a living hell. I can neither give hope to others nor can I take it away. However, if you and I can offer the smallest spark of hope to someone with cancer, then perhaps it will provide that person with the courage to face another day and persevere through their adversity.

Hope then, can constitute many essential elements to the quality of life for the individual cancer patient. Realizing that it is a process, establishing hope in our lives creates a positive outlook for the future. Hope also provides us with a real and/or concrete understanding of our disease situation. Hope also helps us to emotionally connect with others in similar circumstances. Finally, hope in this sense provides us with the background and ability to share our experiences with cancer and offer learning opportunities for others.

Of all the human experiences that we encounter, hope is a type of gift for the future and tells us that we are not alone. Our humanity consists largely of our hope for the future. Hope provides us with an outlook toward the near and far future and provides us with critical information about ourselves and our situation that enables us to cope with what is often considered the unknown. Finally, hope can provide us with strength to face the future realizing that our future is largely dependent on what we think, say, and do with regard to hope's presence in our life.

CHAPTER FOUR:

SAYING GOODBYE

LEARNING TO SAY GOODBYE

By
Richard E. Farmer

There is no doubt that the most spiritually, emotionally, and psychologically difficult thing for one human being to do with another is to say goodbye. And this goodbye is not of the type "and I'll see you later" rather it is goodbye forever because I am going to die. At some level, saying goodbye has a variety of meanings, all of which implies that I will soon be gone, and you will not see me or talk to me. Many people from various backgrounds and religious traditions have differing perspectives on this issue. While generally speaking, saying goodbye implies I will not see you again at least in the context of our present relationship. Many of us do hang on to the concept of an afterlife wherein we pray that we will reconnect with that person. And for some of us, this is partly understood as the joy of heaven.

While I am an important memory for you, my presence in your life diminishes greatly over time usually to the point where I will only exist as a memory or a thought and mostly with a positive connotation. And herein lies the dilemma for most human beings. Over time, the individual who we care about, perhaps deeply care about and even love, will fade or dim as a part of our everyday reality. And therein lies the emotional difficulty of grieving and the conflict that it implies as we struggle to combine both the memories of our prior relationship with the harsh reality of the loss of the physical presence of that person in our life.

Being consciously aware that saying goodbye because we are going to die is a peculiar experience. Most of us construct a reality of living that equates to the idea that tomorrow is yet another day. What we have done yesterday or today is part of our past. How we have behaved toward others. The thoughts we have had, the things we have said, and the ways in which we have behaved are generally part of the past because tomorrow is another day to continue thinking, saying, and behaving. However, if the idea of the emanate arrival of our death is realized, the concept of saying goodbye takes on a vastly different set of meanings.

The most obvious cases of a human condition leading toward death would be those who have been diagnosed with incurable forms of disease most notably certain but not all cancers. Depending upon a vast number of health variables, some cancers are not yet curable or even controllable with various forms of treatment including surgery and chemotherapy. While most health providers are competently careful to diagnose the stages of the cancer and establish a treatment protocol built around those stages, some cancers are just not yet curable, and death is likely within a certain set of parameters. Thus, the need for saying goodbye generally falls onto those individuals who face the certainty of death within the context of the treatment plan and the medical evidence that supports the plan.

Referral to another experience for most human beings. While the idea of goodbye is usually just a theatrical experience, for some the actual reality of the need is apparent. Exceptions to the theatrics include a variety of groups of human beings including those who suffer from a medical diagnosis in which death is a certain outcome or endpoint. This does not, however, include those who suffer death in an accidental manner or as a result of political or social conflict or even mental illness or advanced age.

Goodbye implies relationships with others. Spouses, children, siblings, neighbors, co-workers, and the myriad of others who constitute the emotional community in which we live, recognizing the need to communicate goodbye is paramount. It represents a major task which we must recognize if we are to travel the journey from living to dying in a way that is healthful for ourselves and for those others in our psychological community. Inherent to our relationships within this community are commonly understood as forms of love and caring which provide the basis and the motivation to execute the process and achieve the goal of saying goodbye.

My recognition of the eventual need to say goodbye began when my journey with cancer officially began on November 11, 2014. Unofficially it begins in the early fall of 2014 with my complaining of a sore back. At the time I was a healthy 63-year-old husband, father, grandfather, university professor, and psychologist by profession who was currently serving as President of the Maine College of Health Professions. Successful laminectomy surgery provided little to no relief for the ever-increasing back pain.

The most obvious cases of a human condition leading toward death would be those who have been diagnosed with incurable forms of disease most notably certain but not all cancers. Depending upon a vast number of health variables, some cancers are not yet curable or even controllable with various forms of treatment including surgery and chemotherapy. While most health providers are competently careful to diagnose the stages of the cancer and establish a treatment protocol built around those stages, some cancers are just not yet curable, and death is likely within a certain set of parameters. Thus, the need for saying goodbye generally falls onto those individuals who face the certainty of death within the context of the treatment plan and the medical evidence that supports the plan.

Goodbye implies relationships with others. Spouses, children, siblings, neighbors, co-workers, and the myriad of others who constitute the emotional community in which we live, recognizing the need to communicate goodbye is paramount. It represents a major task which we must recognize if we are to travel the journey from living to dying in a way that is healthful for ourselves and for those others in our psychological community. Inherent to our relationships within this community are commonly understood as forms of love and caring which provide the basis and the motivation to execute the process and achieve the goal of saying goodbye.

My recognition of the eventual need to say goodbye began when my journey with cancer officially began on November 11, 2014. Unofficially it begins in the early fall of 2014 with my complaining of a sore back. At the time I was a healthy 63-year-old husband, father, grandfather, university professor, and psychologist by profession who was currently serving as President of the Maine College of Health Professions. Successful laminectomy surgery provided little to no relief for the ever-increasing back pain. Referral to another orthopedic provider resulted in urgent kyphoplasty surgery in an attempt to stop the cascade of vertebral compression fractures.

A biopsy was also taken which led to the diagnosis of Multiple Myeloma cancer. This is a relatively rare form of blood cancer which is at present, incurable and has an average life span of 6 or more years.

Cancer is a complicated disease. It certainly has a distinct physical aspect that runs a gamut from invisible pain to gross disfiguration depending on the type of cancer one has. Our ability to cope balances a deep-rooted change in our lives, always fearing that many people die an early death from it. Physical changes like strength, balance, and stamina can readily affect our daily lives. On a purely psychological level, we learn that we are somehow different from others because we have this disease in our body and acceptance of a changed self-concept can be psychically painful for many. There are many faces to cancer. These faces run a marathon of feelings – from sadness, fear, joy, belief, faith to a myriad of other dynamics. Just the idea of having a disease in our body can, for some, cause a sense of disruption to our self-concept. And certainly, for all cancer patients and their families a change takes place in our psyche that hopefully provides the opportunity for the expression of courage, gratitude, and positivity.

Such expressions of positivity are well exemplified as to how, I will never know, Bonnie managed to support me; realizing that I stood a good chance of dying before turning 70 years old and leaving her as a widow. Her lifelong experiences as a registered nurse, with a PhD in nursing, and now a retired professor of nursing from the University of Southern Maine continues to positively influence my care and quality of life. She is a unique, strong, and loving spouse who was committed to helping me manage the cancer. But that is the type of person that she is. She is a pillar of strength to me and ultimately to the children and family members, always providing the needed support when someone was in crisis over my disease. I am confident that she brought these same qualities to her patients, families, and nursing students. She was determined that this bad, tragic, and fatal news was not going to destroy us. And over the next few days, we worked out a plan to talk with the kids and eventually my brothers and sisters. We even rehearsed how we would explain everything to them and especially how we would need the children's caring and loving support over the months and years to come.

Bonnie was determined that this bad, tragic, and fatal news was not going to destroy us. And over the next few days, we worked out a plan to talk with the kids and eventually my brothers and sisters. We even rehearsed how we would explain everything to them and especially how we would need the children's caring and loving support over the months and years to come. But that is the type of person that she is. She is a pillar of strength to me and ultimately to the children and family members, always providing the needed support when someone was in crisis over my disease.

Curiously, my diagnosis with cancer was also Bonnie's diagnosis. After 47 years of marriage, at the time, based upon an equal relationship, cancer introduced a sense of disequilibrium to our relationship. As with all marital caregivers, what was once a successful relationship based on an ardent sense of equality of feelings, tasks, responsibilities and the like, was now replaced with some elements that can no longer be held due to the gross physical and emotional maladies associated with the day-to-day realities of the cancer. Simply, I could no longer do things that I always did…household chores, acts of remembrance and kindness, intense and daily relationships with our children and grandchildren, participation in neighborhood events, and the like. This does not mean that I could do none of it, rather the degree of involvement was and is significantly reduced because of the introduction of caring disequilibrium into our marital relationship that was specifically designed to mitigate the physical or emotional requirements of the task. Do recognize though that any changes to our relationship were always delivered by my tears which were supported by our bridge of love.

Our bridge of love was deeply developed by my realization that it was time to consider saying goodbye, first to my wife, children, and grandchildren as age appropriate, close friends and several neighbors. While mixed with tears and sobbing I decided that a multi-step process was important. This included preparing the details of the many household tasks that would fall onto Bonnie's shoulders when I passed. The second task was to prepare a "Love Card" outlining my innermost and deeply held feelings about her and our relationship. I also did this for each of my children and my oldest grandchild. Next, I prepared an "Open Letter" to my wife and children in which I expressed my feelings about them and asked for forgiveness for any transgressions I may have "committed" to them in their lifetime. I did also say openly how immensely proud of them I was and how their accomplishments in life so far were outstanding and how proud I am leaving this world knowing that it is a better place because of what they have done. Finally, Bonnie and I worked with our attorney for a review and alteration of our Last Will and Testament so that all legal matters were addressed. All of these items were placed into a lock box in the office with my wife and children knowing both the contents and its location.

The final step, and emotionally the most difficult one, came next. Over a period of months, I met individually with my wife and children. During these meetings, which was interspersed with many moments of crying, sobbing and tears. I explained that I needed to say – Goodbye – and why it was important for me and for them to be able to bring closure to our physical relationship. And, knowing that our emotional relationship will never end; it will always be with them. At my urging, I stress how important it is to let any negativity go and be replaced with the positive aspects of our years together now and forever.

Like any father, I did ask the adult children to assume certain roles with respect to the legal documents. One child was given the task of helping to assume the role of legal advisor and the other the medical or health advisor who in conjunction with their mother and our lawyer would satisfy what needed to be accomplished with respect to the myriad of legal matters that they will be facing. And I urged and pleaded with them to continue to support their mother for the next period of time would be exceedingly difficult for her.

My meetings with my spouse were regular and ongoing. With the exception of my "Love Card" to her, she was aware of each document and its contents. In many instances, she was involved in the construction of the many documents having to do with our financial matters, our long-term relationship with our financial advisor, and close contact with an attorney. One of her important tasks was to make sure that the Medical End-of-Life documents were on file with the medical caregivers so that there was no confusion about what the staff can, and cannot, do at the end stages of the person's life. Her one "assignment per se" was to make the final arrangements with respect to a funeral.

Saying goodbye is perhaps one of the most arduous tasks that anyone is faced with if they are given the opportunity to do so. The importance of this is both practical in that the final details with regard to end-of-life are taken care of, the legal and Last Will documents and procedures are also addressed with the family attorney, and notification of the death is made to siblings, close friends, and others in the community.

Goodbye gives one an opportunity to both 'close the door' and to solidify the deep love and caring so evident between both the dying person and their spousal and familial relationships and others who are of great importance to the dying person. The fear of the unknown that the dying person often expresses – what happens when I die – can be best mitigated through a spiritual relationship with God and a deep and compassionate relationship with the very many people important to us, and most particularly to those to whom we love now and forever.

We choose to live a positive life, to make a deliberate decision to remain positive in the presence of catastrophic disease. We pray daily asking God to give us the strength to choose being positive. And while bad things happen to people, my spouse reminds me daily of the power of positive thinking which provides the basis for living a meaningful life of love, gratitude, and blessings.

Please pray for us.

SAYING GOODBYE

By
David W. Persky

Saying goodbye is not something I really thought of as I began my journey, although it did cross my mind at times when I was in an emotional rut or not thinking clearly. I do not have a "cancer schmancer" attitude as actress Fran Drescher might say. It never was uppermost in my thoughts once I had a strategy to beat the cancer. As many in the medical profession say, about 80 percent of men in the United States will die with prostate cancer, but very few will die from prostate cancer.

But what if I were in the small percentage of men who succumb to prostate cancer?

How would I say goodbye? Obviously, there will be much emotion and conversation as I spend quality time with my wife and daughter up to the time to say goodbye. I would see my siblings and close cousins to have meaningful conversations with them as well. I would try to buoy their spirits and to keep the conversations as upbeat as possible.

While I have not seriously thought about saying goodbye, I have discussed with my family what to do with my remains after my demise. Most conversations have been lighthearted and we each get a good laugh with the various iterations of what to do with "Dr. P" when he has passed. I have often considered donating my body to science to help advance medicine, either training of medical students or for organ transplants. After donating my body for science, my remains would be cremated, and the ashes would be spread out at various places that have been important in my life: my high school in Shaker Heights, Ohio; Southern Methodist University where I earned my bachelor's degree; Miami University where I earned my master's degree; Florida State University where I earned my doctorate; Stetson University College of Law where I earned my law degree; the headquarters of Kappa Sigma Fraternity in Charlottesville, VA (I am a true frat rat and have been involved with Kappa Sigma in many ways since I first joined as a college freshman); and on the campus of Saint Leo University where I spent the final years of my professional career. By the time my remains get to Saint Leo, there will be truly little left to disperse on the campus!

I do know it is not easy to say goodbye. I realized this when I retired from Saint Leo University. I teared up as I presented my last class lectures to my final four sections in the fall semester. I knew at some level I would not be teaching at Saint Leo again, but I never realized how difficult it would be to say goodbye to the students. I got even more emotional when I said goodbye to my colleagues in the faculty and staff at the university. I had a wonderful career at Saint Leo and the kind words and good wishes from the university community touched my inner core and brought me to tears.

The first time I seriously thought about saying goodbye was several years ago when I visited a friend from elementary school who resides on Cape Cod in Massachusetts. I had been attending a seminar at Southern New Hampshire University while my daughter attended a summer leadership program for high school and middle school students at Harvard University. Mary got to tour Boston and attend a Red Sox game with a friend from Tampa. After the seminar, I returned to Boston and we drove down to the Cape to visit my friend Paul and his wife Leslie. One day after breakfast I took a shower and noticed my face was swelling and my voice was "squeaky" and I was not sure what the cause was, but I was concerned. Paul and Mary immediately drove me to the hospital. As I arrived in the ER, the admitting nurse recognized what was happening as I went into anaphylactic shock. Her quick action got me the medical attention I needed for this serious condition. I do not remember much for the three or so hours I was at the hospital, but I do recall lying on the bed in the trauma room with my eyes closed and seeing a bright light. I was not sure what was happening, but I had heard that many people who are nearing death see a bright light. As I lay there seeing the bright light, I began to think that I might succumb to the anaphylaxis. I am not afraid of dying, but at that time, I was not ready to pass on to whatever awaits me after I die. I did have an internal conversation with my higher power while lying on the bed. I remember telling him that it was too soon for me to die and that I had things yet to do in my lifetime. My daughter was still in middle school and had not yet had her bat mitzvah. I wanted to be there for her to share that milestone with her along with other milestones in a young person's life: graduating from high school, her senior prom, attending and graduating from college. And I wanted the honor of escorting her down the aisle on her wedding day and getting to spend time with grandchildren. The experience with anaphylaxis scared me and I assured him he had my attention and I pleaded that I not be taken that day. There were many conversations that I needed to have before I departed.

I recently watched a "30 for 30" episode on ESPN that dealt with the career and untimely death of former basketball coach and commentator Jim Valvano. Jim Valvano was struck with cancer in his back a few years after his North Carolina State University basketball team won the NCAA tournament in 1983. The cancer was aggressive, and Jim Valvano fought valiantly on his journey as a cancer patient before dying in 1993. At the 1993 ESPY awards, Jim Valvano made his last public appearance, but he made a very profound statement about having a good day that I believe is applicable for those of us on the journey to beat cancer. As he put it, to have a good day you need to do three things: take time to laugh, take time to think, and take time to cry. I try to follow this model each day along my journey and I believe it is appropriate for everyone, whether they are a cancer patient or not. I know it will help me when it is time for me to say goodbye.

LOVE, LEGACY AND BEYOND SAYING GOODBYE

By
Bonnie Cashin Farmer

Much of my nursing career included a significant clinical, teaching, and research focus on the fundamental concepts of aging, death, and dying in later life. Thus, I naively thought that I would be well prepared when my aged parents' health became increasingly compromised. My father was beginning to show slight signs of decline when he received a diagnosis of lymphoma cancer, a blood cancer of the lymphatic system. Because he was in overall good health at the age of 84, chemotherapy seemed an appropriate treatment: four months later he was dead. I arrived at the hospital just after he died and in time to hold his still warm hand. I was most grateful.

Seven years later my mother was diagnosed with lymphoma cancer. At the time she was 88 years old, living in an independent senior apartment, confined to a wheelchair, and severely compromised by arthritis and advanced macular degeneration. Mom decided not to pursue chemotherapy and chose palliative care under medical supervision: should her heart stop, a Do Not Resuscitate order was in place. When hospice eventually became involved in her care, I hired a health aide for assisting her with morning and evening personal care. I repeatedly reviewed hospice protocol not to call 911 with the aide should she find my mother unconscious or dead: call hospice first and then me. In my mind and heart, I had planned a good peaceful death for my mom with loving family by her side. On a Sunday morning, the health aide called me to say that she had found my mother dead on the floor of her apartment. I screamed first and then said, "Well, have you called hospice?" There was silence. The aide quietly replied "no" and informed me that she called 911. As we approached the drive to the building, there were two fire trucks out front plus several police cruisers. As we entered her small studio apartment, at least five or more police officers filled the entire space. My mother was sitting upright on the floor with her back against the bed and her disheveled nightgown exposing her "private" body areas. I grabbed a throw to cover her and was gently restrained by one of the officers who informed me that I could not cover her because her death was "unattended." I then called the hospice nurse to come. Mom had most likely suffered a cardiac event during the night. As to having the gift of saying goodbye in the presence of imminent death, "you don't always get what you want." However, I found much comfort that since the time of her diagnosis, Mom and I had the opportunity to spend much loving, meaningful, and even fun times together in preparing to say the final good-bye.

A lifelong friend from childhood did exactly what she wanted as the end of her life drew near. Her four cancers over the course of 15 years, her four arduous and individual surgeries, and lengthy treatments ended when the metastases no longer responded to any treatment. Her approach to cancer always had a sustained and never changing mantra: fight, fight, fight! In her last week, she was "waiting to see" if she could have another chemotherapy treatment. Right up until the day before her death at age 70, she refused to even say the word hospice. I honored her wishes. Much like the elephant in the room, death filled her every space. Continuing to battle cancer remained her chosen path even when her death was imminent. Her obituary highlighted her long and "courageous battle with cancer." For her close friends, not having the opportunity to say goodbye underscored the sadness of her death and what might have been. In her last months and weeks of life, there was no peace, no calm, no acceptance, and no good-byes for our dear friend: just the lasting echo of her battle cry, "fight, fight, fight!"

Using military terms and concepts of battle, winning, defeat, and survivor can create a mindset that cancer is an enemy to defeat at all costs. The National Cancer Act of 1971, a legislative amendment to the Public Health Service Act of 1944, further solidified this war focused approach. With cancer as the second leading cause of death in the United States, President Nixon officially declared "war on cancer." Although well-intentioned, given what was known and not known about cancer at the time, the presence of this war-like attitude toward "beating" cancer became implanted in cancer culture.

For my spouse and I, "battling cancer" just fuels the presence of negative energy. "Battling cancer" can be deleterious to our personal growth, health, and quality of life while living with cancer. His disease is not the enemy. We prefer to better direct our energies toward finding ways toward problem-solving, informed decision-making, doing our best every day to manage his cancer while cultivating a sense of wellness, and making space in our open hearts for all the goodness that surrounds us. My spouse, a former runner and power walker, will frequently muse on his unmet desire to run a full marathon. He also knows that, for the past seven years, each day of living with his cancer is a marathon in of itself: requiring discipline, training, commitment, and resolve to complete a walk across the room, out to the yard, or down our dirt road. We stand with him at his daily finish line, cheering him on and knowing full well that he is an elite runner by any standards. Cancer exacerbates the reality of eventual death. The joyous birth of our newest grandchild has underscored the acknowledgment of the probability of not seeing the baby takes his first steps, say "Papa," or begins first grade. I often ask him how he can be so sure that he will die before me: a wink and a hug usually follow. I find a place for his incurable cancer until a crisis, an infection, a fall, or a "bad lab report" rears the closeness of death once again. In a health crisis, we wonder if this will be "it", the fever, the infection, the hospitalization, the continued loss of weight chops away at us bit by bit. "It" is always in the back of my mind: his impending death.

Almost immediately after his cancer diagnosis, my spouse and I updated our Advance Directives, implemented an immediate No Chest Compressions Resuscitation order and became familiar with burial options. The life decisions we now make reflect living with an incurable disease. We live with saying good-bye in both direct and indirect ways: some more subtle than others. He has created several files of financial information, household vendors, and home maintenance information to "assist" me with tasks that I have done successfully for decades. I appreciate his loving efforts. He continues to worry that I have yet to learn the protocol of filing federal taxes. He has written letters, for family and close friends, to send upon his death. He has comprised a list of persons with contact information who "might want to know" when he dies. His detailed efforts reflect his enduring love and care for his family.

As of today, my own cancer has not placed me within an urgent need to say goodbye or at least I do not think so. Last year the bevy of tests looking for metastases as cause of unexplained weight loss brought the reality of my own cancer experience into a sharper focus. I find myself expanding my provenance for the children, cleaning out items that I know for certain that they would not want. I continue to work on marking some items as to their origins with any stories that may accompany them, identifying valuable items not for a dumpster, and starting a jewelry list of what I wish for whom. Last Christmas, during my many diagnostic tests, my daughter laughingly mentioned how much she always loved the two-little vintage Santa figures on the mantle and could I please put her name on them. I felt good that we can have these conversations. We continue discussions with the children about an equitable system for dispersing our home and its contents. Our wills are clear and protective trusts are in place for them both.

As my parents aged, I recall them doing similar things like periodically showing me where to find their wills and important papers. They arranged their burial plots years before their deaths. As an only child, I was their one heir. I did not want to be an heir. I just wanted my parents. I would tell them that I did not want to hear "it." "I," being when they die. One day as my parents were preparing to move out of state, my dad asked me to store a large-framed picture of his mother at our house. I regretfully was a little short with my reply as to where I would have room. He looked pleadingly at me and asked, "Please?" To this day, the picture remains in my basement among my family treasures. I have curated my own memorabilia to include those which are most meaningful to me or might be welcomed by our families. I also know full well that many of my "basement treasures" will likewise be disposed of when I die. I accept that such treasures have meaning only to me: my first-grade class picture, a decayed movie stub, or the disintegrating flowers from my wedding. Legacy is so much more than obvious possessions.

More important than any plastic crate of "treasures" is my eternal legacy of the always and forever love for my family. My life's tapestry will eventually become a woven part of each family member's own tapestry: will live on within them as our family members before us have done. To this day, I find myself repeating my mother's phrases and hearing Dad's laugh on my shoulder as he shakes his head saying, "Oh, Bonnie!" I look for a recipe in the little wooden boxes filled with Mom's hand-written recipes and I feel her presence. I carry on the annual Christmas traditions such as making Mom's stollen and putting money in the Salvation Army's red bucket. When the grandfather's clock in the dining room chimes, I often think of it as Dad saying, "hello." Prior to her death, my mother-in-law gave us the beloved Christmas dishes that we had given to her decades before. She wanted to be sure that we had them. Each year when we take the dishes out on Thanksgiving Day and put them away on Valentine's Day, I always whisper a thank you to Grammy for giving them to us. The thank you is not just for the dishes. The thank you is for her love for us.

My family, deceased and alive, all contribute to who I have been, am, and will become for as long as I live. Death will not end the long and full life that I have been blessed to share with my spouse. Amid grief and sorrow, as our boundless love for each other transitions to a different form, may our hearts remain open for the joy that we so cherished together. My spouse and I will be cremated upon death. Initially we thought an individual burial would follow. However, we have decided to save our ashes until the time that we can be buried together; nothing less will do for our forever and always love!

THE PINK ELEPHANT

By
Cherie LaFlamme Genua

Two days after my course of radiation ended, my dad passed away. He did not die of cancer, but of heart issues that worsened in the months leading to his death. I remember feeling so many emotions that week—from the highest of highs to the lowest of lows—including happiness, sadness, guilt, pain, sheer exhaustion, and a glimmer of hope for my own future. I was beyond thrilled that my active treatment was coming to an end. After six months of chemotherapy, surgery, and thirty straight days of exhausting radiation, I closed that chapter of my journey. Then, my dad died, and my emotional state dipped down into a deep, dark place.

All I could think about was death and endings.

Before cancer, death was a sad and depressing term. I remember how badly my eyes stung from crying out of sadness after losing both of my grandmothers over the years. One grandmother died suddenly during a rather routine operation, while one died over several weeks in the hospital. I cannot be certain, but I think she knew she was dying. My family and I definitely knew she was dying, but I never really said goodbye. I ignored it like the pink elephant in the room. Instead, I made small talk with her to lighten the mood. We watched episodes of I Love Lucy as life support helped her breathe. I watched in sadness as she wrote phrases in a notebook because she could not speak any longer due to the tracheotomy. I tried to be upbeat and strong because that is what I thought she would want from me. Looking back now—after facing my own mortality at the age of 34—I would have handled things differently when I knew it was time to say goodbye.

Much like my grandmother, many terminal cancer patients know they are going to pass away. They, perhaps, do the work internally to face those fears and they get to a place of acceptance. Loved ones sometimes take the path of ignoring or distracting from the fact that they are probably going to die. During visits with that person, we concentrate on anything and everything besides the cancer. We will talk about the weather or a movie we we just watched. We will reminisce about a trip we took together in college or the time we went to New York City to see that Broadway play. These conversations are great to have, of course. And even though the topic of their mortality might feel off-limits, it is just as important.

These days, if I knew that a friend or loved one was going to die of cancer (or any terminal illness), I would ask if they wanted to talk about it. If they wanted nothing to do with my suggestion, I would avert my attention back to the television or the card game or whatever else we were doing. If they agreed, though, I would put my phone down and clear my mind. And most importantly, I would listen. Asking the question - "do you want to talk about it?" - gives them permission to share their thoughts and feelings. To the person with a terminal illness, it might be a relief to address dying in a concrete way: they might not feel as comfortable bringing it up out of fear of upsetting you.

A conversation on death and dying might naturally morph into a conversation about the life they lived and the memories you shared. Write down or record the special moments or stories you do not want to forget. You will never regret snapping more photos or capturing a video clip of your loved one's voice to listen to later. You might regret, however, not capturing those same moments. I often think about the wisdom my grandparents shared with me over the years. I wished I wrote down anything and everything. I wished I asked more questions about their youth and their experiences. There is no right answer to bring up death or reflecting on a full life of memories, but having the conversation should tell them that they are important to you and that you cherish their words and feelings.

I would imagine that some people who know they might die might want to talk about the parts of their lives that they regret. They might even want to apologize for some things. Listening while having an open mind and heart is all you have to do—there are no magic words or phrases. Life is complicated. I think if my dad knew he was going to die when he did, he might have apologized for some of the things he put me through. And I would have forgiven him because a lot was beyond his control.

I am comfortable with the topic of death now. However, being in remission, it is difficult to talk about how I would feel if I were to say goodbye to my loved ones, particularly my husband, my mother and stepdad, my extended family, and my cherished friends. I feared death early on in my diagnosis, but that lessened with time as I started treatment. Even though I am not in a place where I am saying goodbye, there are still areas in my life that I strengthened post-diagnosis to help me live life to the fullest:

- For starters, I found comfort in my support system of friends and loved ones. They cheered me on through treatment and talked to me when I was having bad or scary days. They made me feel loved every step of the way. I also found it important to make sure my family and friends knew how important they were to me, too, because we never truly know how long our time on this planet is. My main priority for the rest of my life is to ensure the people closest to me know how important they are to my heart and soul.
- This leads me to my next point: always knowing what is important. For me, the most important things are my family, my friends, my Portuguese Water Dog, seeing the world, enjoying the breeze from a nearby body of water, and otherwise being in nature. These are the things I cannot buy from a store, of course.
- I found support through other cancer survivors. Cancer is a lonely journey at times, no matter how many people you are around. Finding comfort and strength through other cancer survivors or support groups helps because you can openly share your feelings and experiences with others who are facing similar challenges. No matter what stage of a cancer journey, fellow cancer patients can be key in coping with and working through complex emotions.
- I pray—plain and simple. Having a higher power to talk to about my deepest and darkest fears help me work through things and makes me feel at ease. Even if you are not religious, finding spirituality can lead to a sense of calm and comfort.
- I wanted to learn and create! Work was always a part of my identity before I became ill. I still enjoy the work I do, but I find joy in other ways now, too. I take free online courses to learn new subjects. I finally put ink to paper and wrote the fiction novel I had on my mind for years. This new love of learning and creating is something I hope stays with me for the rest of my life.

- Giving back and volunteering became top of mind. There are always people less fortunate than us, even when we are dealing with a cancer diagnosis or terminal illness. Being gracious and giving to causes that you feel passionate about can make a world of difference in your mental state. Laugh—at yourself, with others, and everything in between. Your sense of humor during a crushing time in your life is something that can carry you far. Laughter is the best medicine and it's free. I put up a photo of my bald head on social media wearing a green face mask and laughed at the absurdity of it. I did things I never thought I would do, but it made me feel better.
- Lastly, do not be so hard on yourself. Cancer is hard. It is not easy physically and it is even harder mentally and emotionally. I had days where I cried out of sadness and fear in the shower. I felt like my body had failed me when I could not get out of my bed for days on end. But I always remembered that better days were coming and I would not feel like that forever. If my body needed rest; I gave it rest. If I needed to cry and splash water on my face in the second floor bathroom at work, that is what I did.

Getting diagnosed with cancer hits you like a ton of bricks. It does not matter the type, or stage, or prognosis. No one wants to hear those words. It inevitably forces us to consider our own passing, whether we want to think about it or not. Those with a cancer diagnosis—or those who know someone who has died from cancer—know all too well that people die from this disease. It is why we cry when we hear that diagnosis because it's oftentimes associated with death and dying. Of course, many of us go on to live long and fulfilling lives after a cancer diagnosis, but it undeniably makes you think about how we live and what is important.

And for those people with a more terminal illness, saying goodbye means looking back and also looking forward… perhaps on the milestones and memories that they might miss out on should their time on this planet come to an end. But what if we look at the flip side? Tomorrow is never promised, no matter if you do or do not have cancer or another terminal disease. Some people die suddenly without the opportunity of true reflection. In some ways, I see the ability to look back and reflect on one's life and purpose to be a gift that many people do not get to experience. None of us know what tomorrow brings and many of us will not get to say goodbye. All we can do is live our lives in a way so that if we are ever faced with saying goodbye, we will be proud. Proud, perhaps, that we did not wait until our final days to relive and remember the most precious moments over the course of our lives and pleased, maybe, with how we did not hesitate to tell loved ones how important they are and will always be.

RINGING THE BELL AND SAYING GOODBYE

By
Burt Harres

Nowadays, it seems that nearly every cancer facility has bells that patients can ring to mark the end of treatment. It is believed that this tradition began at The University of Texas, MD Anderson Cancer Center, in 1996. A rear admiral in the U.S. Navy, Irve Le Moyne, was undergoing radiation therapy for head and neck cancer and told his oncologist that he planned to follow a Navy tradition of ringing a bell to signify "when the job was done." He brought a brass bell to his last treatment, rang it several times and left it as a donation. It was mounted on a wall plaque in the Main Building's Radiation Treatment Center with the inscription:

Ringing Out
Ring this bell
Three times well
Its toll to clearly say,
My treatment's done
This course is run
And I am on my way!

Some cancer patients ring the bell more than once because their treatments involve a combination of surgery, radiation, and chemotherapy. Other patients' cancer may return and require additional treatment.

The American Society for Radiation Oncology has reported that a study published in the International Journal of Radiation Oncology * Biology * Physics revealed that of a survey of 200 patients with cancer, half of whom rang the bell at the end of treatment and half of who did not, found that those who rang a bell remembered treatment as more distressful than those who finished without ringing a bell. That outcome surprised the study's lead investigator, a radiation oncologist who led the study while completing his residency in California. "We expected the bell to improve the memory of treatment distress," he said. "But in fact, the opposite occurred. Ringing the bell actually made the memory of treatment worse, and those memories grew even more pronounced as time passed. We think this is because ringing the bell creates a 'flashbulb event' in a patient's life – that is, a vivid snapshot of their memories from that time," said the radiation oncologist. He further explained that events become more deeply embedded in our memories if emotions are aroused, due to connections in the brain between memory and emotion. "Rather than locking in the good feelings that come with completing treatment, however, ringing the bell appears to lock in the stressful feelings associated with being treated for cancer."

This practice of "ringing the bell" has received criticism from some patient advocates who note that there are other patients whose treatment may not end on a positive note or only end upon death. For these patients, hearing the bell ring can arouse an array of feelings such as anger, resentment, depression, or despair since they will not likely be given the option to ever ring the bell. Ringing the bell is also a very personal decision and will vary among cancer patients. Each cancer patient is encouraged to consider the pros and cons of this practice before deciding if it is right for them.

Ringing the bell could be considered by some cancer patients as a form of saying goodbye to cancer. In my journey as a cancer patient, I decided not to ring the bell because I never considered my battle with prostate cancer to be over. I view my battle with prostate cancer to be on a continuum. I continue to have annual examinations by my oncologists that include blood analysis, body scans, and transrectal ultrasounds. I avoided ringing the bell because, although it is considered a well-intended practice, it was not one in which I needed to confirm the successful milestones of my cancer treatment. I also did not ring the bell to "celebrate" my milestone if it would have any adverse effect on other cancer patients who heard the bell ring but whose prognosis was not as favorable as mine and who may never have the opportunity to "ring the bell."

In my case, thanks to the early detection of my prostate cancer and outstanding treatment by my oncologist, the ongoing reports I received about my condition were always favorable. Consequently, I never considered developing plans to say goodbye within the context of my cancer. However, I was involved with my father's process of "saying goodbye."

In June 2006, my father was hospitalized because he was experiencing difficulty in breathing. I was in Orlando, Florida for a one-day professional conference when I received a telephone call from his doctor. Much to my shock, he informed me that tests confirmed that my father had stage four lung cancer. I was stunned because my father's lung cancer had not been previously diagnosed and for it to have become this advanced left me speechless. My father's doctor told me that most lung cancers do not cause any symptoms until they have spread, but some people with early lung cancer do have symptoms. I asked him when he would join me in telling my father that he was diagnosed with lung cancer. To my dismay, his doctor told me that I could inform my father of his condition by myself and that he did not need to be present. In retrospect, I should never have agreed to comply with the doctor's directives. My father's doctor should have been the one to inform my father that he had cancer and to answer any questions about my father's treatment plan. I should have been present and at my father's side to offer my love and moral support but not to provide medical information. Unfortunately, I was not thinking clearly after receiving the terrible news about my father's diagnosis. My drive from Orlando to the hospital in Crystal River, Florida was terribly sad and seemed to drag out forever. When I informed my father of his condition, we hugged and wept. It was one of the saddest moments of my life and as I write this sentence, I am still choked with tears.

A couple days later, I returned to the hospital with good news to share with my father. I had just been promoted to the position of vice president of instruction/provost of the West Campus of Pasco-Hernando State College. My father's formal education ended when he graduated from high school so when he heard of my success a broad smile crossed his face. I remember him saying, "Burton, I'm very proud of you. Just remember to never act like a big shot." "Never act like a bigshot" became my personal mantra.

My father was a resident at an assisted living residence in Crystal River. It was there that he entered hospice care. I remember visiting him on the Fourth of July 2006. He was connected to an oxygen tank but was in excellent spirits. We enjoyed a lunch of barbeque chicken, coleslaw, and baked beans. He was excited that his brothers (my twin uncles) and my two sons (his grandsons) were going to be visiting him next week. Since my uncles would be in town, I had planned to attend a Volunteer Florida

Commission meeting in Palm Beach: being gone for a couple of days seemed feasible. However, the day before I was supposed to leave for the meeting, I had a feeling come over me that I needed to stay home. I canceled my trip.

On July 9, 2006, my uncles, my sons, and I visited my father. He seemed to be very happy. We talked for hours and reminisced about bygone days. When we were about to leave, I gave my father a kiss on his forehead like I had done countless times. I remember standing at the doorway to his apartment and saw his smile evaporate from his face to be replaced with a look of calm.

On July 10, 2006, my uncles, sons, and I returned for another visit. Upon our arrival, we were informed that he had recently entered a coma. We stayed for about an hour and decided to leave my father since he was "resting". None of us realized or were informed by the hospice staff of the severity of his condition.

At approximately 2:00 a.m. on July 11, 2006, I received a call from a nurse at his residence informing me that my father had passed away. Later that day, I spoke to the director of the assisted living residence and told her I felt awful that I was not with my father when he died. She told me that she learned over the years that many of her residents had voiced their wishes that they pass away alone while asleep instead of having family members by their side. She said that my father held on to see his brothers, my sons, and me one more time before he "let go." To some extent, I still feel anguished that I was not with my father when he took his last breath. However, I am comforted in knowing that he said "goodbye" on his own terms.

Nevertheless, for those cancer patients who are or will plan on saying goodbye, I offer the following information developed by the American Cancer Society. According to the American Cancer Society, preparing to say goodbye at the end of life is not easy, and often does not come naturally. It also may be hard to do because of a patient's health status, capacity, or where the patient is receiving care. Every person's situation is different. No one can really predict what may happen at the end of life, how long the final stage of life will last, or when death will actually happen.

The American Cancer Society offers the following suggestions that may help you and or your caregiver(s) in planning to say goodbye at the time of end of life:
- Try to plan ahead, but remember it is not really possible to predict when the last hours or minutes of life may happen.
- Understand and respect that each person has different needs and ways to express how they are feeling...
- Be open about knowing the end of life is approaching is.
- Try to avoid topics and unpleasant memories that may cause hurt, stress, or pain.
- You do not have to be formal with goodbyes when taking a b r e a k from being together, or if a caregiver is leaving the room for any reason, just expressing your love is often recommended by hospice experts.
- Consider other types of communication for people who may be out of town or traveling, such as phone calls, video applications such as FaceTime, Skype, or other technology.
- For caregivers, know that many healthcare experts believe those who are unconscious or unresponsive may still be able to know you are present and can hear what you are saying.

The American Cancer Society is an excellent resource for helping the cancer patient and caregiver(s) make these very personal end of life plans.

To state that saying goodbye at the end of life is not easy is an understatement. Saying goodbye at the end of life can be unthinkable. Planning for saying goodbye ahead of time before the end of life can potentially provide all individuals with a way to clarify decisions regarding care for themselves should they no longer be able to make such decisions themselves. Multiple reliable resources for Advance Care Planning can be accessed online through physicians, hospitals, government sites, or through healthcare organizations and community health programs.

As I recall the last days of my father's life, I would be remiss if I did not mention the importance of an advance directive. My father was very thoughtful and had advance directives prepared. My father's advance directives ensured that his preferences regarding his end-of-life health care would be honored by his family and health care providers. His preferences were contained in a legal document known as an advance directive, that would only be effective if he was incapacitated and unable to speak for himself. My father's advance directive consisted of a living will and durable power of attorney for health care (sometimes known as a medical power of attorney) that he had prepared by an attorney years ago. Advance care planning is not just about old age. My father realized when he was healthy that planning for health care in his future was an important step toward ensuring that he would receive the medical care he wanted if he was unable to speak for himself. My wife and I have advance directives. I strongly

recommend that everyone, regardless of their age, have advance directives.

According to the American Cancer Society, the living will is a legal document used to state certain future health care decisions only when a person becomes unable to make the decisions and choices on their own. The living will is only used at the end of life if a person is terminally ill (cannot be cured) or permanently unconscious. The living will describes the type of medical treatment the person would want or not want to receive in these situations. It can describe under what conditions an attempt to prolong life should be started or stopped. This applies to treatments including, but not limited to dialysis, tube feedings, or actual life support (such as the use of breathing machines).

A durable power of attorney for health care, also known as a medical power of attorney, is a legal document in which you name a person to be a proxy (agent) to make all your health care decisions if you become unable to do so. Before a medical power of attorney can be used to guide medical decisions, a person's physician must certify that the person is unable to make their own medical decisions. The person you name as a proxy or agent should be someone who knows you well and someone you trust to carry out your wishes. Your proxy or agent should understand how you would make decisions if you were able and should be comfortable asking questions and advocating to your health care team on your behalf. Be sure to discuss your wishes in detail with that person. You may also choose to name a back-up person in case your first choice becomes unable or unwilling to act on your behalf. Durable power of attorney laws vary from state to state: meaning the state in which the individual is present and receiving care. Talk to your health care team and check the state laws.

At this point in my journey as a cancer patient, I offer the following lessons learned:

- Ringing the bell, like planning to say goodbye, is also a very personal decision and will vary among cancer patients. It is advisable and important for a cancer patient to consider the advantages and disadvantages of this ringing the bell before deciding if it should be incorporated in their treatment plan.
- To state that saying goodbye is not easy is an understatement. Each cancer patient will have to determine if and how he or she will plan on saying goodbye. The American Cancer Society is an excellent source for helping the cancer patient and caregiver(s) make this very personal plan.
- Having an advance directive can be extremely beneficial, as it allows you to specify your wishes while easing the decision-making burden on your loved ones. Advance directives can provide clear guidance to health care providers, reduce the likelihood of a dispute with and among family members, and ensure you avoid unwanted procedures. Making sure that your doctors, hospitals, and all relevant persons have the most recent copy of your advance directives on file remains an all-important requirement for the implementation of your decisions.

Lastly, saying goodbye reflects the end of our physical presence on earth. And, for many persons, saying goodbye can also reflect the transition to the afterlife for the deeply spiritual.

CHAPTER FIVE:

A MEANINGFUL LIFE

LIVING A MEANINGFUL LIFE

By
Richard E. Farmer

Living a meaningful life has many definitions or ways of understanding the concept. At first glance, it implies how we spend our days thinking, doing, interacting and has some intrinsic meaning to ourselves and others. Meaning, of course, implies that there is some internal or external value in what we say or do. While this typically involves other people, meaning or meaningfulness also has great internal or intrinsic elements for each of us individually or just within our own self. And when combined with a focus on other people, we have the ability to best understand what the idea of living a meaningful life is all about. The intention of this work is not only applicable to cancer patients per se, elements presented here have inspired reflection for all of us. What follows are some ways of thinking about the effects of cancer on us with respect to meaningfulness as well as examples that all of us face as Cancer Patients.

Regardless of where you are in the progression of cancer – newly diagnosed, in therapy, in remission, and even cured, you will most likely think of yourself as a cancer warrior who has fought a battle and has won the war! You are victorious as you have braved the dreadful and scary enemy that medical science calls cancer. The cancer label we attach to ourselves stays with us for our lifetime and becomes a sort of veil under which we view others, our experiences, our family and loved ones and ultimately the world. This cancer veil in a sense uses a key which we turn to understand ourselves and our experiences both positive and healthy, and negative and personally hurtful. And, with effort and learning to understand consequences, we can turn the key in any direction to move the veil to yield a different consequence or outcome.

The cancer experience has the possibility of making the individual self-oriented versus other-oriented. And while there are many reasons for this happening, cancer can easily and readily make one self-absorbed because the disease involves virtually every part of the physical and emotional make-up of the individual. Loss of perspective and consequently loss of hope in the future, obsessive reliance of medication for a cure, and the loss of touch with one's feelings, friends, and even family are common experiences for the cancer patient, especially in the early phases of the disease. And while time will help mitigate this because of the seriousness of the disease and the idea that it never goes away and is only dampened somewhat over time. Hence, the idea of the creation of the Cancer Patient.

There is little doubt that everything in one's life changes when diagnosed with cancer. All of a sudden you are confronted with the idea that you have a disease which could be and in fact is fatal for some. This will cause you to redefine your role as a person, spouse, friend, lover, parent, grandparent, worker and professional, neighbor, and the like. The added dimension of cancer into the mix of statements that define us creates an imbalance. And this imbalance adds a dimension of facts, feelings, thoughts, and ideas that we have never had to deal with in the past. This is to suggest that the diagnosis forces us to redefine our roles ranging from the most intimate and familial to the more casual.

Redefining your role or who you are requires that you incorporate your cancer into all aspects of your being and the various roles that you play. This is not playing as in game playing, rather it is the relationship with yourself and others including the physical, emotional, and psychological aspects of who we are as a person. Prior to our diagnosis, cancer was not an element of this although declining health most likely a part, and the one which drove you to seek medical attention in the first place. You now have cancer, and that fact occupies a significant or even major part of who we are as a person. This major part requires us to incorporate our "new identity" as an individual with cancer as an element in everything that we do.

As this new identity becomes widely known or public knowledge, we encounter shifting sands no matter where we are. Unbelievable, it would seem, that everyone we encounter knows that we are ill with cancer. And what most people do not know is that while some cancers are incurable and fatal, not all cancers are this way. Yet, many will look at us and talk with us asking how we are feeling and if there is anything that they can do to help. They generally do want to know our status and are sincere about their willingness to help. However, some lack an expression of empathy toward us and will "write us off" as friends or acquaintances because we may make them uncomfortable because they fear that we will soon die, forcing them to deal with that fact.

Children, siblings, and other family members are an entirely different matter. For most, at the heart of our family relationships is love. Above and beyond all else, love provides a type of vehicle that provides special access to our inner being. This access enables both the family member and the cancer patient to be exceptionally open and honest about the individual's experiences. While this is not universally the case as some patients may hide information about their cancer as a means for 'protecting' the family loved one from the harsher realities of the disease and its treatment. And, as one might expect, this is especially true for harsher therapies including surgery and radiation and the later side effects.

All of this said, familial love is a powerful source of comfort for the cancer patient. Being present and highly empathic, expressed love can help us to feel calm and cherish their presence in our lives in person, on the telephone, or through the internet. Feeling connected is especially important for the cancer patient precisely because we are so potentially disconnected from other elements in their life. And, as the disease progresses with either cure or death as the end outcome, love from family during the process is especially comforting and therapeutic.

Spouses are an incredibly special category both in terms of love and their degree of importance to us. Clearly, it is the spouse that plays multiple roles with regard to the cancer patient. In addition to the normal or typical spousal roles, the spouse commonly assumes caregiver duties which help the patient to manage medical appointments, treatment drugs and pharmacy relationships, and other aspects of helping the patient to better manage their disease. Spouses are soul mates to the patient often experiencing many of the disease-related activities required for the cancer treatment of the patient. It has even been suggested that in a highly positive love situation, both the patient and the spouse have the cancer because the role of the spouse is to fill in the palliative gaps missing from the medical treatment of the vast array of other effects which are caused by treatments of varying types. Ultimately, spousal love helps to treat and maybe even help to treat or cure the individual's cancer.

It is important to point out that being a cancer patient is often seen as walking through shifting sands. How we define ourselves, and how that definition translates into our relationships with friends, co-workers, family, spouses, and others will change over time. The sands do shift with respect to the type of treatment we receive, its success, our managing side effects and the glowing light of a possible cure or death as appropriate to our disease. Change is the operative word that describes who we are as cancer patients and the other people who play a significant role in our lives. Preparing for that change as we go along in time is critical to the successful management of our disease.

Over time we will experience changes in our disease, in our relationships with friends and co-workers, employment, family and spouses. The analogy is like we will experience 'cloudy weather' from time to time. Expectations about the progress of our disease can and will change as it is likely not to meet our expectations, our interactions with the oncologist and palliative care physician can be helpful one meeting and challenging at another, our children may from time to time be unable to meet our emotional needs or even occasionally treat us with a sense of callousness when we expect warm and loving responses, they may even 'bug' us with annoying questions about the status of our health or how a particular appointment with our physician went, and pour spouses may constantly and sometimes obsessively monitor our behaviors which do or do not follow the prescribed course of action. Please know that these cloudy weather situations are only temporary and occasional. Nonetheless, we need to prepare ourselves emotionally for their occurrence.

Despair is a common feeling or sense of self as one begins the long process of dealing with their cancer. Despair may be seen virtually over everything in what can be considered as a former life. Everything has changed including our work, even our finances, our friends and neighbors, our recreational activities and exercise patterns, our relationships with our children, siblings, extended family, and naturally our spouse and our patterns of intimacy. "How did this happen?" "Why me?" "What did I do to deserve this terrible disease?" The answers to these and many other questions are not readily answerable, although some may be obvious like heredity or occupational exposure. And because of this lack of a clear cut or defined answer to the "why," despair may set in for many of us. Unless dealt with, despair for some may turn into forms of mild to severe sadness or if left unresolved, depression or even in more serious forms of psychological distress may set in.

Another routine form of life for the cancer patient lies within navigating the choppy waters of our existence. Meaning that most of us have good and not-so-good days. Most of this, but not all, is attributable to our cancer situation. That is, while every human being travels with choppy water of good and bad and up and down as we go through life, cancer adds an additional albeit unique dimension to our experiences. This means that the cancer itself, the medications we take to deal with the disease and side effects, radiological or surgical treatments undertaken, and our emotional state because of it contributes in a meaningful way to our state of being. And because of this, we are somehow or somewhat different people than we were before diagnosis. "Okay, so I've had enough" say some cancer patients when they realize what has been happening to them as a result of the disease. What follows then are many options or ways of positively dealing with the disease so that we can add meaningfulness back into our lives. One way of thinking about this is that the cancer diagnosis and subsequent treatments can add up to a "new birth" of ourselves. Recognizing that yes, we are different now, is an important first step when we add to that further statements that indicate we are still okay, that we are still good and wholesome persons, that we still love and are loved by others, and that we will deliberately choose a positive path for the rest of our days which are filled with hope.

Assuming that our particular situation with respect to meaningfulness is part of the tapestry of one's life, there are very many things that can be done to improve our situation. First and foremost, it is important to form a team that will help you to navigate the multiple details your healthcare providers require. Much like each of the members of your local football squad, each team member can and should have a role to play that will assist you in scoring the point by achieving your particular goal. All cancer patients readily understand the complexity of their disease corresponds to the complexity of the number and roles of healthcare providers assigned to your case. For most of us, this is initially burdensome since rarely is there a navigator to help us understand the complexities of the medical staff who will assist us in managing our case. So, form a team of individuals who can help us to keep track of the requirements and suggestions of the medical providers. Typically, this team is composed of spouses, and/or adult children, and unusually maybe even friends or neighbors who are willing to take on the responsibility of membership. Be sure to record or keep notes about appointments, questions, answers, directions, orders for forthcoming medical appointments, pharmaceutical needs, and related information. The team and your notes will definitely help you to keep track of the sometimes fast-moving items to accomplish or at least be aware of. Finally, just remember that little things do count!

Some things to consider with respect to the use of our "team" and how we deal with issues post-diagnosis. Some of this is just attitudinal and some just practical. We need to find a way to deal with those choppy waters. Some things to also consider with respect to the use of our "team" and how we deal with issues earlier. With the help of our team, we can find a way of creating calm amidst the chaos of the moment. We can draw a line in the sand indicating that you've had enough, you can put out fires in your life that popup suddenly because you have the strength to do so. You can create a new normal in your life by deliberately choosing to do something or not. Finally, you can choose not to fade away over time by being diminished and deliberately not involved.

With respect to family, it is incredibly important that they be included in the process of information sharing. Sometimes we develop the mistaken belief that we do not want to burden them with the facts about your disease. After all, our adult children and perhaps siblings have their own lives to lead and worry about and are usually or typically filled with the normal stressors and strains of adulthood. However, your silence or failure to 'tell the truth' about the aspects of your disease only serves to add to the stressors and strains currently experienced by your adult children. And, for your not-so-adult children, acceptable versions appropriate to their age is also acceptable and necessary. And, as we know, children and family members of all ages are highly perceptive and will come to their own conclusions regardless of the accuracy. Also, if grandparents are part of the family composition, it is important to specially include them in information sharing realizing that this may be a significant source of stress for them.

Friends are an especially important group of people who care about you and who generally want to help in any way that they can or that you allow them to. Many cancer patients believe that their medical status is their business, and theirs alone. That is, they do not wish to share this information with these friends for any number of reasons. Keeping this information silent is potentially hurtful to a trusting friendship because many cancers affect us in ways that are obvious to others, especially those who know us well. In the end, we must remember that our friends do care about us and would absolutely want to help in any way they could. Also, we may well need the assistance of our friends to help us to do things that we are temporarily unable to do. And friends are excellent sources of people who care about us and would readily serve as individuals with whom we can share our thoughts and experiences with the disease. Friends have ears and they can help!

Like most of us, cancer patients may need to hone their skills of gratitude. Family members and friends who go out of their way to call us or send us get well cards or emails must be thanked either by you assuming you are well enough to do this or by a team member if you are unable to do so. Meeting individuals in public who express their concern for us also requires us to give an appropriate response. The idea here is that outside of our immediate family, there are many people such as friends, neighbors, and acquaintances that will express their concern for us and we need to be able to warmly thank them for their interest and how that makes you feel with a sense of gratitude.

Your attitude is an especially important source for adding meaning to your life. How you view certain situations that you may find yourself in will determine for better or worse how it will affect you attitudinally. And the old adage about bad attitudes creating bad outcomes is certainly a perspective to be aware of. For example, using the "H" word or the Happy word is an attitude perspective that can help us to rethink or reanalyze situations that we may find ourselves in. Too, espousing hope about a situation or even the future clearly puts us in a better frame of mind than does the opposite which only suggests fear. Another attitude common among many of us facing difficult situations such as being a cancer patient is to not be afraid to ask for help. For some, our disease may have placed certain limitations upon our abilities to accomplish things. And while we have always been able to do them before, we may now find ourselves in a situation in which we are physically unable to complete a task. In this instance, asking others for help is critically important, even though it somehow goes against our prior life experiences and can only be accomplished with the assistance of others.

There are any number of examples that all of us could identify that are indicative of the new person we are becoming because of our cancer diagnosis. You are asked to engage in a personal reflection after each of these two vignettes or brief statements about the new meaningfulness in your life:

1. There is a recent example of a male homeowner who is facing the end of the Fall season and the burden of cleaning rain gutters has usually been his responsibility. Even though this individual has many physical defects and muscle problems as a result of his cancer, he brought out the step ladder and climbed it only to discover that it was not long enough to assist him in reaching close to the top so that he could reach over and clear the fallen leaves. Damn he thought, I used to always be able to do this: anger and frustration seethed through his mind.

Knowing that winter would soon be upon them, what would you do? Obviously screaming, yelling, raising your fist to the sky was not going to solve the problem. The solution was to go out and purchase a slightly longer ladder. And yes, it costs some money, but being able to avoid the anger and frustration is far more costly in the long run.

2. A middle-aged female homemaker was an avid gardener during the spring and summer seasons. Her yard and home abounded with beautiful flowers and plants: she was the envy of the neighborhood. Having recently had a double mastectomy, she often worked lightly in the gardens and it was a wonderful way for her to engage in the healing process. Realizing that her garden work was extremely helpful to her physical and emotional healing, she decided to make a major addition to one whole side of the garden in the backyard. She put on her garden clothes and gathered her many tools and went to work.

Her first chore was to dig out a large strip of lawn to make room for the new flowers and plants. She started digging and digging and digging and within a truly short period of time totally she became exhausted and completely frustrated. She sat on the ground and burst into uncontrollable tears when she realized that it would be unlikely that she would ever accomplish what she wanted so very badly to do. Picking herself up and off the ground, she decided that further crying was not going to do anything but make her unhappy, sad, and frustrated.

So, she could either hire a neighbor teen or use a landscape service, or even choose a different project that she could readily accomplish. Remaining angry and depressed about her changed health situation was of no value in adding further gardening pleasure to her life.

Triggers are situations or events which when we experience one which causes a particular emotional reaction in us, most commonly anger is the reaction. Meltdown is a common trigger that creates a strong emotional anger reaction and can easily help rob meaningfulness in your life, if only on a temporary basis. Meltdowns are triggers that rob us of meaning especially when there are many triggers in our life. Understanding what those triggers are can help us to find alternative modes of behaving and thinking that will neutralize its effects upon us or even add to our overall life's meaningfulness.

One final source of difficulty especially aimed at cancer patients is the idea of who is minding the store? Meaning that we have the probability of a quagmire of healthcare providers and places of treatment. This can be highly confusing and a source of stress and confusion when you combine the totality of cancer-related providers, our personal care providers for non-cancer health care, dentists, pharmacists, and other responsibilities of living and the like makes most of us keep a detailed notebook/calendar that allows us to know what we need to do on a daily or weekly basis. Clearly, our team can help us keep track of the very many things that we are required to do.

There are very many things that we can do to increase the level of meaningfulness in our lives as cancer patients. These will include:

- Recognize that we are multidimensional people versus singular. This means that we are more than "just" cancer patients
- Recognize the more common problems of cancer patients: obsession with medication, lack of hope for the future, loss of touch with your feelings, friends, and family can isolate us from those very people in our lives who love and care for us and make us feel isolated.

- Becoming self-versus other oriented. Because cancer typically involves every part of our physical and emotional self being, we tend to focus on ourselves forgetting that there are other people in our lives, and we need to find a way to incorporate them into our thinking and behavior. Ask others for help, you must remember that you are not by yourself in your cancer journey.
- Draw a 'line in the sand' meaning that you will only go so far and not any farther in dealing with the multitude of issues typically faced by cancer patients.
- Create your own 'new normal" which tells you about what you are and are not any longer willing to do. This can also be communicated to others.

Living a meaningful life is important for all of us and is especially important for cancer patients. As all cancer patients know, the disease will quickly destroy meaning in one's life as we attempt to cope with an all-encompassing disease. Understanding this process is vitally important for the successful treatment of the disease. We need to come to terms with the fact that cancer has changed much about who we are; it robs the prior meaning we had about who and what we are, at least to some measure. Bearing-this-in-mind, we have the knowledge and ability to reach within ourselves and recreate who and what we once were. Recognizing that meaningfulness is the cornerstone upon which we rebuild our lives post diagnosis is the very first step in this process. Good luck!

MEANINGFUL LIVING

By
David W. Persky

As noted earlier, I retired from Saint Leo University before I received the diagnosis of prostate cancer and began my cancer journey. Two major shifts in my life altered my notion of a meaningful life but I have reflected on this idea quite a bit during my journey.

Early in my professional career I had a conversation with one of my mentors who shared his thoughts on our place in the world. He believed that we are trustees for the world we find ourselves in at any given time. As he explained it, we hold this world in trust and our role is to make it better for those who follow us. This idea resonated with me and it was a guiding principle for me in my career as a faculty member, as an attorney and as an administrator. I believe it is the essence of living a meaningful life.

I spent the majority of my professional career in higher education in both the public and private sectors. For a short period of time, I also practiced law in Tampa. Shortly after I returned to Tampa, after completing my doctoral studies, I had the opportunity to join Civitan International, a service organization that was founded in Birmingham, Alabama in 1919. The club that I joined was an interesting mixture of university staff members and residents from the communities around the University of South Florida. Civitan has been known around the country for one of its preeminent programs, the sale of Claxton Fruitcakes. That was not my reason for joining and I have done my best to distance myself from fruitcakes, except to play Jimmy Buffet's song "Fruitcakes" during my term as District Governor. I was attracted to Civitan because of its motto, "Builders of Good Citizenship" and the many local service projects we undertook to help make our community better and the opportunity to give something back to the community. I have volunteered with the Florida Special Olympics at the state, regional and county level for many years since joining Civitan. I find it most rewarding to work with the Special Olympics to help the athletes and their families. The pure joy and happiness on the faces of the athletes is to me, the epitome of living a meaningful life.

Another of the most significant examples of a meaningful life for me came early in my legal career. I have been a volunteer attorney for the Volunteer Lawyers Program of the Bay Area for more than 30 years, starting as a third-year law student in a Civil Clinic internship in the 13th Judicial Circuit in Tampa. Clients are seen on a pro bono basis. The first client I met with was a woman who was experiencing significant financial troubles and had lost her job. She was on the verge of being evicted from her home. I spent time with her reviewing the various options available to her to find a new place to live and other job opportunities that might provide new employment opportunities for her. We see clients in similar situations at almost every intake session but what made that session so meaningful was the client was extremely grateful that I would spend time with her and actually listen to her problems and provide some options to help her get back on her feet. I happened to see her approximately six months later working at one of the stores in a local mall and she had been able to turn her life around with some of the information I was able to share with her.

The positions I held in academia provided numerous opportunities to interact with students, faculty, and staff, and in many instances to make a positive difference in their lives (and continue to live a meaningful life myself). I did not always realize the impact(s) I made on students and others initially. And I did not show up at work each day with the idea of seeking a situation that I could get involved in to improve the lives of people that came to see me that day. But in each term situations would arise, and I would do what I could to assist and achieve a positive resolution for the individuals involved. To me, it was part of my job to assist the students (or staff members) who sought me out.

Some were easy to resolve. I could make a call (or calls) to the appropriate office to refer the student so he or she could get the assistance or guidance they needed. On some occasions, I had to contact other attorney friends to provide legal counsel to help student(s) in various legal disputes, both criminal and civil. In many situations, the assistance I could render was a response to the person who contacted me with a legal question. While I was not the general counsel for the university, many faculty and staff thought I was their attorney, regardless.

When I retired, I assumed that I would no longer lead as meaningful a life as I had while working with and advising students and colleagues at Saint Leo. But so far, I have found that I am able to live as meaningful a life as I did before retirement. Former students and staff members have reached out to me for assistance in applying to law school or graduate school or to ask for letters of reference as they sought jobs in their chosen professions. It is particularly meaningful to hear from former students who recognize that the legal concepts studied in my courses gave them a competitive edge over their classmates in law school.

I know I am able to provide guidance and counsel to other prostate cancer patients who received their diagnosis later than I did. Paying it forward for others is another way to lead a meaningful life. I have learned that it is possible to continue leading a meaningful life beyond my active working career and to help make the world better for others who will follow.

NAVIGATING CHOPPY WATERS

By
Bonnie Cashin Farmer

Some three years ago on a bright and sunny summer day, my spouse and I were riding with our daughter and her family on their boat. The very effort of getting their beloved father and Papa onto the boat proved to be a bit tricky but they did it. Seated in a camp sling-like chair, my spouse was comfortable and secure. We were both delighted just to be on the ocean water with the family! The wind began to pick up during the afternoon and the waters of the bay became increasingly choppy. The ride became very bumpy. Our hats were off or lose them forever. In place of our usual non-stop family chatter to which we are so accustomed, we all sat quietly heading back to the dock.

As the water churned and the wind blowing on my face and through my hair, I closed my eyes. Sitting very still, I became filled with a sense of joy and peace of the present moment. It was a wonderful feeling! I then heard our daughter's voice, "Mom, Mom are you okay?" I opened my eyes. She asked if I was feeling sick from the rough waters. I reassured my precious child that I was not sick and just enjoying the moment!

The idea of experiencing joy and peace amidst chaos and disequilibrium on our now "forever" choppy waters provide a conceptual foundation for my sharing of living a meaningful life in the presence of my cancer with vigilant surveillance and my spouse's incurable cancer. Admittedly, I have always been partial to metaphors for better understanding of certain phenomena. Decades ago, long before the practice of mindfulness became popular for many, I became interested in the concept of "nowness": …being in the here and now… yesterday is past, tomorrow is in the future. A little paperback text in my bookcase, now tattered with yellowing pages, provides a gentle reminder of the importance of living in the present moment. My spouse and I have not just been holding steady on choppy waters; we have been living, and living well, within our given circumstances.

Our circumstances for my spouse are challenging even on a "pretty good day" and excruciating during crises. We acknowledge that if today is "pretty good" then today is as good as it will ever get for us. If only internally, I, for one, have chosen not to dismiss these "pretty" good days. "No regrets" has been my driving goal for not wasting "pretty good days" with terror of all the unknowns of tomorrow! Dwelling upon the future can negatively detract from our present "pretty good" here and now. At times we even thrive amid day-to-day uncertainty. I take it in, I deal to the best of my abilities, and I let it go whenever possible. Being and living in the here and now is not easy.

With all that said, I have also found that the common phrase of living every day as if it was your last, is not sustainable. About a year after his diagnosis, my spouse mentioned how much he would love a blueberry pie. I recall vividly that it was a Saturday evening about 7:00 pm. At that point I had not even entertained the idea of creating some caregiving boundaries to sustain myself and immediately began making a pie by 7:15 pm. I truly was not thinking clearly as evidenced that I had never been a pie maker! I was blindly driven by my need to make him happy. Although he was not in crisis at the time, my motivations included thinking what if this would be his last pie? I was still trying to make the pie 'til late that evening while he had long gone to bed. The next day, as he enjoyed his blueberry pudding, we both realized that living every day as if today was our last day together was not living in the present moment. Feeling the love between us every day as if today was our last is easy.

Much like the variability of choppy waters, the underlying presence of sadness is a constant. Although our sense of overall loss of quality of life could be paralyzing and allow little heartfelt openness for anything else, our blessings are abundant and at times even overwhelming as we cultivate our capacity to experience them. I had never embraced the idea of the gifts received from my spouse's or my cancer: "gifts" seems like a superfluous word to describe how cancer has impacted our lives. However, I suspect that the periods of my spouse's extended periods of being critically ill have influenced and shaped our acceptance and gratitude for the gift of living a "pretty good" life. Living in periods of health crises can rapidly put being "okay" in perspective. We choose to be positive while acknowledging our circumstances; being positive is a choice. For us, choosing to be positive is not denying our circumstances nor being unrealistic. Some days are harder than others. Tomorrow is uncertain. We then dust ourselves off, let it go to the best of our abilities, and nurture an open heart.

I find it interesting how individuals can be seduced by the false sense of certainties. No one ever lives on certain ground. Nothing about life is certain other than as sure, as the sun rises in the morning and sets at night, all human beings eventually die. The diagnosis of cancer forces an up close and personal reflection on the certainty of dying. Accepting death as a certainty of the human condition comes the freedom of opportunity to shape one's life. I am not always successful, yet peace does come with continuing to do my best while accepting that I am human and imperfect. The waves of choppy waters are always moving and in flux: big, little, rough, or rogue. Keeping a steady course is a goal and not a destination.

Living with my spouse's cancer eventually has become a way of life for us. I am not implying that I like it, I never asked for it. I fervently wish that our life in our later years had been different. We eventually embraced deep within our very souls that this is our life as it has unfolded: a life never asked for, nor desired. Once we stopped trying to maintain normalcy as we had known it, day to day living began to gradually improve. We turned a corner in optimizing our being: becoming grateful for what we can do given the circumstances of my spouse's debilitating disease. Being present, really present, is a gift to those you love.

Our loving relationship never included keeping a scorecard but rather a quiet balance of life upon which we both had opportunities to thrive as individuals, as a couple, and as parents and grandparents. Now that balance between us as we knew it is no longer. This sustained imbalance demands constant attention and readjustment of focus and expectations by both of us. My spouse has struggled with adapting to his limitations and accepting what he can and cannot do; watching me struggle with certain tasks is tortuous for him. Early on, one of the first times I left him on his own for a brief time, I came home to find him trying to climb a very shaky ladder to fix a light bulb! He no longer climbs any kind of ladder. We continue to work in a positive direction toward developing an attitude of acknowledging limitations and embracing what we have and what we can do.

The basics of everyday living require attention even in the presence of cancer. Having the capacity to identify and communicate what is possible and what is not has allowed our life to become more manageable. I feel grateful that I have the physical capacity to complete new-to-me household tasks. My spouse is less grateful about learning how to separate clothes before washing and folding laundry. After a blizzard with a snow accumulation of 17 inches, I checked the drifted snow by the garage door before going to bed; the garage door would not open. I immediately went out to shovel before the plow came. My spouse became upset and yelled, "why are you so determined to shovel by the door now?" I realized at that moment that there were lots of reasons with one being able to open and access the door in the event of an emergency or needing immediate transportation. Upon reflection, I finally realized that I was also doing it because I am very fearful that I cannot do it. I am driven to be confident that I can do what needs to be done and take care of both of us: admittedly sometimes to a fault. This experience led to many insights of how I was and was not addressing my own physical status. Just because I could shovel by the garage door did not mean that doing so was in the best interest for my body.

Most of my physical limitations, present prior to my cancer diagnosis, are now exacerbated by aging and the cumulated side effects of oral adjuvant chemotherapy with an aromatase inhibitor. With some adaptations and modifications, I can manage most of the necessary indoor and outdoor household and garden tasks. With a keen eye for safety, I will often look for new ways to reduce strain on my body. For example, I quickly replaced our heavy and narrow-step ladders with lightweight aluminum ones with wide step platforms and a secure standing area. Last summer, when we had a new tree planted in the front yard, a two-wheel hose truck (yes, that is the correct term) for watering became my best friend! Thinking through the best way to efficiently accomplish a task, before I do it, has proved helpful and hopefully more sustainable.

Time management for me remains challenging at best. Time seems to evaporate with a blink. Unanticipated issues for my spouse, some more serious than others, can occur with much frequency and can require time-consuming interventions. For example, medication side effect du jour, unannounced periods of incapacitating fatigue, infections, health insurance denials and approvals, ever-changing food preferences, new prescriptions, and infections could make a "pretty good life" miserable. Prioritizing my time is essential toward nurturing a "pretty good life' and maintaining a relatively steady course even in the presence of rogue waves.

Prioritizing my time also includes making some kind of emotional space for myself. Despite retiring four years ago, I soon found that occasional lunches with friends, a day trip to the botanical gardens, or a walk on the beach just took too much time away from home. Since there is so little extra time on any given day, I thought about how I might cultivate this personal space within our "given circumstances" meaning: remaining at home. Since music has always been an important part of my life, be it listening to music or making music with a clarinet or a violin, I decided to take out my beloved guitar and see what would happen. Despite my ever-present desire to play the guitar, I never did learn how to really play it. Three years ago, I joined a local community folk ensemble taught by a professional teaching artist. One hour, one day a week, plus at home practice times of my choosing, has taken me where I never could have even imagined. Playing my guitar fuels my soul and makes some wonderful moments and experiences
within a "pretty good life".

Since my high school days, I have always found inspiration in the poem, Desiderata (Ehrmann, M., 1927). As a teenager, I would ask to read the poem as part of prayer and grace for holiday dinners. My desire to read the entire poem while the food became cold eventually led to pre-dinner recitations. This poem then became part of our wedding ceremony and incorporated within our children's wedding receptions. I frequently harkened back to the last line all of the poem:

With its sham, drudgery, and broken dreams,
it is still a beautiful world.
Be cheerful. Strive to be happy.

I continue to weave my life's tapestry with unlimited threads of all colors, sizes, and imperfections: unique, individualized, and all my own. Throughout this ever-expanding tapestry, among the more prominent and reoccurring deeply woven threads are living a life of genuine gratitude. I often wonder how my adoption influenced this sustained presence of gratitude in my life. My children, even when they were young, still recall me saying, "my cup 'runneth' over with blessings." On occasion, they still will ask me, "Mom, is your cup running over?" My reply to this very day is always the same, "yes."

Several years passed from my spouse's diagnosis when, for the very first time, my spouse said with profound tenderness how sorry he was for me that he got cancer. I acknowledged his feelings and heard and felt his angst. I asked how he would feel if our circumstances were reversed; knowing well that he would do the same for me. Brief and poignant discussions ensued about how much we love and have loved one another for 50 years. Therein lies the heartbreak and the joy. In the words of Kahlil Gilbran (1923), "The deeper the sorrow, the greater the joy." Joy can seep in where the seeds of sorrow are sown. Nurturing our capacity to experience the snippets of joyful moments or more in each day (most of the time) has contributed to living a meaningful life. For example, a few years ago as I was standing at the kitchen sink, I had a mini epiphany: if my spouse had not been forced to retire due to his cancer, he and I would still be working! There would not have been an occasional movie or a lobster shack luncheon on a weekday afternoon nor our new ritual of a daily glass of wine at 5:00 pm with engaged conversation prior to our dinner.

With my deliberate creation of emotional space for the experience of joy, however brief or fleeting, grows an openness and peace of heart. Over the decades of my life, I have made many attempts and much progress, two steps forward one backward, toward I do not know exactly what. Yet I acquiesce that cancer has allowed me to "arrive" and find my voice without apology: confident in expressing what I think, what I do, what I feel, and who I am. I have peace of heart knowing every day, I continue to do the absolute best to my abilities in navigating our choppy waters. I will remain forever grateful.

MOVING FORWARD

By
Cherie LaFlamme Genua

Learning how to live again after treatment was daunting. I thought that this chapter of my life would slam shut and I would be able to pick up and resume life as it was before my cancer diagnosis. But it was not that easy. I found it hard to resume my past life. As much as I did not want to be a person with a cancer diagnosis; I did not want to be the person I was before my cancer diagnosis either. I was a changed person, after all, with different priorities and a new outlook.

All cancer patients and survivors have completely different experiences (which is so very evident in this book). One thing is universal, though. Cancer forces us to be introspective as we think about our lives. It is up to us—and us alone, really—to live a meaningful life after a cancer diagnosis.

But the question is: how do we do that?

I spent a lot of time in nature while I was recovering from treatment. I wanted to get exercise, of course, but I also found the outdoors to be comforting. It was the perfect place to think about what was next for me. I recall one summer morning when I went for a hike in the woods near my house. My face was warm and flushed and my bald head was sticky from the heat. I sat on a rock and removed my hat for some relief. I stared at my surroundings and took it all in. I inhaled the fresh air and shut my eyes as the rays from the sun grazed my skin. I was still. And I was ready to face my fears.

It was on that rock that morning where I let go of a lot of anger that I have been harboring since my diagnosis. The "why me" questions nagged at me behind the scenes of my otherwise positive exterior. Yes, I had a brave face and I moved forward, but I couldn't help but be a little bitter. But, right then and there, I did my best to let it go. As much as I blamed myself, getting cancer was not my fault. It was up to me to take something positive out of an otherwise negative experience. So, that is what I did. I exhaled the negative thoughts and feelings about my diagnosis and treatment, as well as the events or moments that I missed out on. I inhaled a future full of health and wealth—not in money, but in the things that were a priority to me.

Cancer has a way of showing us what is important in life. It becomes clear very quickly that material things are not at the top of the list. For me, the special people in my world—my husband, my family, and my close friends—and the time spent creating moments with them are what became important. I began craving experiences with my loved ones... the types of days I would remember for the rest of my life. I relished in the big and small moments. There were days that seemed average to most, where my husband, dog, and I would get in the car and drive to a wooded spot to go for a hike. But to me, those moments started becoming so necessary and cherished. Walking in the open air at my own pace outweighed the thrill of buying a luxury vehicle. A birthday celebration that consisted of a "paint night" with a glass of red wine and laughter became far more special than a diamond necklace. Putting my phone down and watching the waves roll in and out on the Connecticut shoreline was my idea of peace and happiness. And it did not cost a thing. A cancer diagnosis creates an appreciation for life and the time we have. The small joys of life take on a new meaning and become sweeter.

This is not to say I lived recklessly before my cancer diagnosis by any means. I was satisfied with life and my purpose, but I felt like I prioritized different things. I was driven and passionate about my career and was always connected to my phone or laptop. I found fulfillment in climbing the ladder at work and taking on more and more. I moved around the country in my 20s for jobs and traveled frequently. The next step, I thought, was to earn an advanced degree in the hopes of getting to the next level. And I did—I finished my MBA months before my cancer diagnosis. But, as soon as I heard those three words—"you have cancer"—my dreams of climbing the corporate ladder took a back burner. My main focus turned into taking baby steps towards healing and health.

During treatment, my only goal was to get through each day. I tried not to get frustrated with myself. On days when I was very fatigued, I rested. Even if I did nothing that day aside from getting out of bed to get a glass of water and a meal, I did not count it as a failure. On days when I woke up and decided there was no way I could work, I stayed home. I learned how to take care of myself and listen to what my body needs. This also goes for days on which I was feeling good. I forced myself to take walks or get out of the house to get some fresh air and distract myself. Although I felt accomplished when I had a great day at work or a fun outing with friends or family, I tried my hardest not to get down on myself when the only thing I could do was turn on the television and haphazardly watch an episode of a show. All of it—the good and the bad days—were critical in my mental and physical health.

It was the time between and after treatments that I found to be the most introspective. It is when I thought about my life before cancer and what I wanted my life to look like in the future, as uncertain as that may have been at the time. What was my life's purpose? What was I meant to do or otherwise accomplish? Did I even know myself as much as I thought I did? I searched for meaning everywhere I could find it—on the rock in the woods, on walks around my neighborhood, and on the couch as I watched the willow tree outside my window sway in the breeze. My thoughts started to become vulnerable. I thought about my life in my 20s and 30s and how confident I seemed to be as I breezed through without much care. But thinking back on my pre-cancer days, I realized I was far from confident. I was searching for something that was not there and I was not sure what mattered or made me happy. Yes, my friends and family were a constant part of my life, but I found myself lacking satisfaction.

While I was not happy to receive a cancer diagnosis by any means, it was not until I got diagnosed with cancer that I was able to see my true self and find the happiness and confidence I'd been lacking. I started to change things about myself that I was not happy with. For instance, I stopped comparing myself to other people. With social media and everyone sharing the happiest—and sometimes, not authentic—parts of their lives, it is hard not to compare yourself to others. During my cancer journey, I shared real, raw, and emotional photos that I never thought I would in a million years. Photos of me with blotchy skin and no hair or eyebrows. But I am positive that those photos and vulnerable posts helped people understand my journey. I also believe they provided strength to those who might have been struggling.

Turning a negative experience into something positive became important to me as I completed treatment. Nothing felt more critical than focusing on my own health and well-being: mentally, physically, and emotionally. Seeking help in the form of support groups and therapy became top-of-mind in my survivorship journey. There are so many emotions and fears to unpack following a cancer diagnosis or at the end of treatment. I felt bad discussing these emotions with family and friends, especially because I did not want my own fears weighing on them. Finding a group full of people with similar journeys or talking to an objective therapist allowed me to say what was on my mind without the worry of making my loved ones more afraid than they already were. I also learned that therapy is not a one-size-fits-all situation—it is truly trial and error. One support group might work very well for you, but it might be a terrible fit for someone else trudging through a cancer journey. The same goes for therapy. And that is okay—if we try and it does not feel right, we owe it to ourselves to be honest with the other party (whether that be a therapist or a support group) so we can move on to something that does feel right. There is always someone out there willing to help and lend an ear to listen or advice to give… all we have to do is find them.

Mental health is critical to living a meaningful life. One of the things cancer survivors dwell on is its recurrence. Being mindful of the risk of recurrence, while also not allowing it to consume our thoughts and happiness, becomes critical in our well-being. During a "survivorship care plan" meeting, my oncology team went through signs and symptoms to look out for in relation to recurrence. That conversation was stressful. I already felt like every new pain or twinge was related to my cancer. But then I thought more about it—it is good to be educated and mindful about your body and what to look out for without letting it overtake our livelihood. Our medical teams are looking out for us with regular appointments and scans, and no amount of stress or sleepless nights can prevent a recurrence. The best we can do is manage the stress and follow the advice of our medical teams by living healthier and modifying the things in our lives that we can control (like physical activity, limiting alcohol, watching what we eat, etc.). Stress and worry will eat us alive if we let it.

When I was close to finishing treatment, my best friend and I joined our other two friends on a trip to Barcelona. We walked the city streets for miles on end, stopping only for a glass of wine (moderation!) or a tapas-filled lunch. We talked and watched people walk by without an agenda. We visited the Sagrada Familia and prayed as the light from the stained glass windows cast colorful reflections across our faces. We marveled at the sights and sounds all around us. We enjoyed each other's company. Not only did the stress seem to lift off of my shoulders, this trip allowed me to live in the moment. I did not worry about the mess I left at home or an upcoming appointment with my oncologist. Instead, I enjoyed the company of my friends and did not fret about the extra money I spent on vacation. While going on trips is something I will always prioritize, it is not for everyone. At the time, I was fatigued by immunotherapy and my stamina was low, which is why I was grateful my friends did not mind a slowed-down trip. You might have different activities that bring you joy and reduce stress. For example, doing yoga in the park, planting vibrant-colored flowers in your garden, or visiting a museum or landmark that you have been wanting to see. Those are examples of small joys that may bring happiness and open the window into a meaningful life. It is important not to allow activities or trips that should bring joy to otherwise make you frustrated or sad. Stick to small or otherwise attainable pleasures and live in the "now." As my oncology team always says to me, "Take it one day at a time." This goes for active treatment, follow-up appointments, scans, and remission. Enjoy every day, because tomorrow is never promised—this goes for everyone, not only those suffering from a cancer diagnosis.

As a cancer patient, we learn that life is the most precious commodity there is. My cancer diagnosis taught me that living a meaningful life was the key to my healing as I moved forward. I turned my bitterness into gratitude for being alive and for having people in my life that cared deeply for me. I began appreciating the small joys of life, instead of taking them for granted. I found happiness by nurturing my physical and mental health and letting go of any resentment I was harboring. Learning to live life again after cancer was one of the toughest parts of my journey. It is also the part that has brought me the most fulfillment as I continue to learn about myself and my purpose. I have a feeling that this is only the beginning of the meaningful life I am meant to live.

HAVING A MEANINGFUL LIFE

By
Burt Harres

I imagine that like many people, there are certain moments in life that are unforgettable. For those of us born in the early 1950s or in prior decades, we can recall where we were when we learned that President John F. Kennedy was assassinated, when Neil Armstrong first stepped on the moon, or when Henry Aaron broke Babe Ruth's home run record.

For me, one of life's memorable events was October 30, 2012 when I was informed by my urologist that the results of my biopsy indicated that I had prostate cancer. Many societies and religions use notations to label or number years such as BC (Before Christ), BCE (Before Current Era), CE (Current Era), and AD (Anno Domini). I suspect that for many cancer patients, time is also bifurcated into the notations of BCD (Before Cancer Diagnosis) and ACD (After Cancer Diagnosis). God has blessed me with a wonderful life, during both BCD and ACD periods.

I was born and reared in a small, agriculture-based community, Columbia, Illinois, 30 miles southeast of St. Louis, Missouri. My early years were spent on a farm with my father and grandparents. Although my parents were divorced when I was four years old, I never considered that I grew up in a "broken home" but rather one in which faith in God, love, and respect flourished. Columbia was an idyllic town where "everybody knew and looked out for everybody." I attended small elementary, middle, and high schools where I had an opportunity to actively participate in athletics and theater. Although I was an average student, with much support from teacher and mentors, I became the first generation of my family to attend college. I then pursued graduate studies which culminated in earning a Doctor of Philosophy (Ph.D.) in Higher Education Administration.

My career as a higher education administrator, serving in various administrative capacities in numerous college and university settings, spanned five decades from 1976 until 2014. Upon my retirement from Pasco-Hernando State College, the District Board of Trustees granted me the title of Vice President of Instruction/Provost Emeritus. I am presently an adjunct instructor of humanities at Pasco-Hernando State College. I also work part-time at a golf club and compete on the Golfweek Senior Amateur Tour.

Like most people, my personal life has had its good and troubled times. I was divorced twice. My first wife, Louise, and I have two sons. The older son and his wife have made me the proud grandfather of four grandchildren. Louise and I remain friends. For almost seven years I have been married to Marilyn, who is the love of my life and best friend. I am the stepfather to her adult children. As Roman Catholics, our faith in God is a very important quality of our lives. I know my faith in God and the power of prayer provided me with the strength I needed and continue to want as my journey as a cancer patient continues to unfold. Marilyn and I serve as Eucharistic ministers at our church.

It is ironic to me that for the last several months prior to my writing this chapter of my journey as a cancer patient, I have been reflecting on the meaningfulness of my life. I have been examining and strengthening my faith in God. I have also viewed YouTube videos and read articles about strategies for developing a meaningful life. I have tried to differentiate between a happy life and a meaningful life. I have determined that happiness involves being focused on the present, whereas meaningfulness involves the past, present, and future and the relationship among them.

In many ways, I have tried to merge rather than separate the BCD (Before Cancer Diagnosis) and ACD (After Cancer Diagnosis) periods of my life. Cancer altered my life, but it does not define it. I refuse to accept a victim mentality. I have come to embrace the concepts for a meaningful life advanced by David Loker, co- founder of WaveAI, Inc. Locker provided the following suggestions for a meaningful life in an article that appeared in Lifehack.org:

- Know what is important for you. Identify the top five things that you believe are the essence of how you want to live life.
- Pursue your passion. Pursuing your passion in life is what makes life worth living and gives our lives true meaning and purpose.
- Discover your life's purpose. If you had to give yourself a reason to

live, what would it be? What principles do you hold highest?
Be Self-Aware. Remain mindful of what you do at all times, and make sure you are living according to your principles, your life's purpose, and what you are passionate about.
- Focus. The world can be very distracting. Try and stayed focused on your primary goals rather than chase a multitude of goals. Not only will you alleviate some of the stress associated with trying to juggle so many tasks, you will be much more successful.
- Spend money on people rather than things. Think about spending your money on experiences with family and friends. Not only will this give deeper meaning to your life by focusing on relationships rather than material wealth, but you will be a happier person as a result.
- Live with compassion. In the words of the Dalai Lama, "One must be compassionate to oneself before external compassion.
- Find a way to give back. Do something that both honors your beliefs and passions, while giving something back to the world.
- Simplify your life. By simplifying your life, you will have more time to do what fulfills you and gives your life meaning.
- Establish a daily list of three goals that adhere to your set of principles and beliefs. By trying to do less, you will wind up doing more.

Accomplishing all these suggestions at one time might seem daunting, but you can pick one suggestion at a time and slowly incorporate these concepts into your life.

At this point in my journey as a cancer patient, I offer this final set of take-aways:

- Although cancer will alter your life, try your best to not to let cancer define your life.
- Life is a journey. Living a life of purpose gives both fulfillment and meaning to your journey.

EPILOGUE:

LESSONS LEARNED

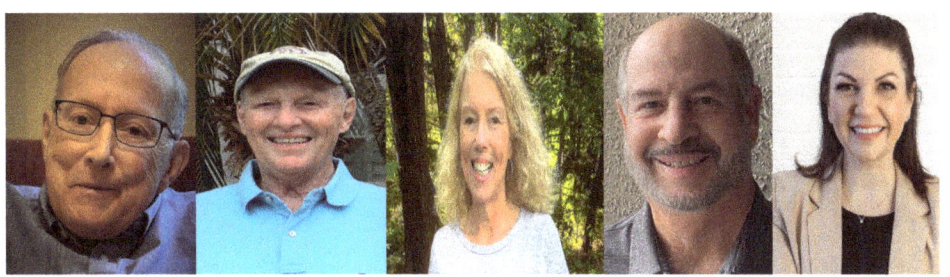

As the reader is aware, this book is the result of the experiences of five individuals as they have coped with a cancer diagnosis. Richard E. Farmer is the senior author and determined the five topics that each author was asked to write about. Thus, there are five common themes or topics that each author has written about. The Epilogue attempts to review what each author has chosen as the most significant Lessons Learned. To this extent, what follows represents their story as a result of their reluctant cancer journey.

Richard E. Farmer

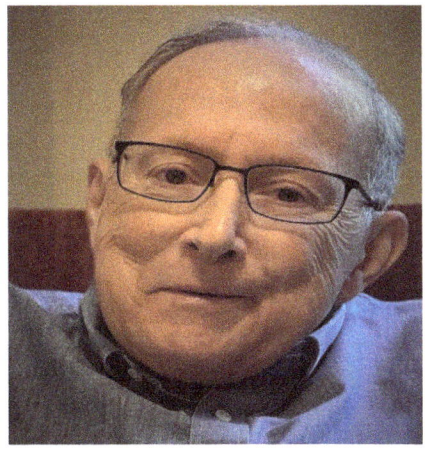

From a significant perspective, I identified "Being A Cancer Patient, Saying Goodbye, and Living a Meaningful Life" as the set of the most important topics presented for me. In general, I determined that these topics best described my view of the core of living with cancer. Articulating the development of Multiple Myeloma and its effect on myself, my spouse, children, grandchildren, and siblings represents a powerful alteration of my personal, familial, and professional core sense of self. Understanding these effects upon myself as an individual and upon virtually all others has helped me to garner a more comprehensive understanding of the role of the cancer diagnosis in my life. As reviewed, this understanding began with the effect of the diagnosis on my physical being and the resulting psychological experience. Recognizing that these two elements can and did play a significant role in my now developing sense of self was important in my ultimate recognition that the cancer diagnosis changed me. These changes created a different person than had been present before. And this difference has had both positive and negative consequences and viewpoints as one examines me prior to and after diagnosis. The idea that one must be prepared for these positive and negative changes is critical to the successful adoption of these new role behaviors as they affect us internally with our own self-concept and externally with our behaviors involving other people.

My coping with individual conversations on a sustained basis with my spouse and family to discuss my diagnosis, treatment, and likely prognosis referred to in terms of end-of-life and saying goodbye is a significant aspect of my cancer experience. Without a doubt, perhaps the most difficult aspect of adapting to a role that includes the concept of death is a realization that the cancer role may include an understanding that one's death can be an integral part of the role. This is not to suggest that all cancers have a terminal outcome. In fact, many if not most cancers are curable. However, the idea that one needs to have a discussion with loved ones and others about one's death is but a practical expectation that others will hold for us.

Saying "goodbye" is a process fraught with emotional trauma regardless of its presentation of one to the other. Saying goodbye to loved ones and others because of an anticipated death requires a coping ability beyond that which is normal. Understanding the intimate nature of one's role is necessary in order to have a successful understanding outcome involving the cancer patient and single people of meaning so that the conversation can be built around the concept of love. And it is the concept of love that is the critical outcome of all discussions involving one's potentially anticipated conversations about death. And the final importance of this discussion is not that death is per se certain, rather the reality of potential cancer death is far more realistic than other forms.

My commitment to "Living a Meaningful Life" represents a commitment to living a life built upon faith and love. No matter how much time we are blessed with, the idea that we will commit ourselves to a meaningful life is critically important. Newly diagnosed cancer patients eventually conclude that they have two paths of living and perhaps more. We learn that we have the path of grace, willingness, commitment to others, love, caring, and the desire to bring meaning to our lives and that of others. And yes, the alternative is that we can isolate ourselves and complain about the tragedy that has befallen them with their diagnosis. Ironically, the cancer lifestyle can prove to be fulfilling and meaningful to ourselves and others around us. We are given the opportunity to make the decision about which direction we shall take. And for me, cancer has taught me to reach beyond myself in order to best encounter others directly and indirectly and hopefully make a difference in their lives.

David W. Persky

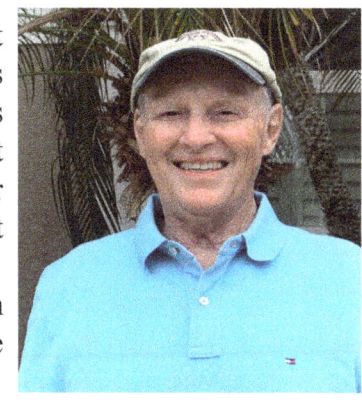

My reluctant journey as a cancer patient has taught me that the fight against this disease is a multi-faceted battle that brings many challenges. I have tried to present some key points to consider helping other cancer patients on their respective reluctant journeys.

As I have written and revised my section of this book, I have spent a lot of time contemplating the most significant lessons learned on this journey. I had not really given the topics much thought until Richard Farmer asked me to contribute to the project. As I reflected on my journey, I recognized three of the topics as being most important for me.

"Being a Cancer Patient" provided me the opportunity to consider the impact it has had on my life. It has shown me how fragile life truly is and how quickly a seemingly healthy person can have their life turned upside down with the receipt of a cancer diagnosis. It upended my life as I transitioned from full-time employment to retirement. I was challenged by the diagnosis, but I did not let it take away my positive approach to dealing with and beating the cancer. I have realized that cancer can "happen" to anyone and that it does not alter the essence of who the patient is. It becomes another fact of life that you, the cancer patient, must deal with. Rather than wallow in self-doubt or pity, remain upbeat with a healthy outlook on the illness and the challenges ahead. My mantra was "Let's go kill some cancer" each day I went for radiation therapy and during the ongoing ADT and it has helped me successfully overcome the obstacles of prostate cancer. You are stronger than you may think you are and with a positive outlook, you can beat the disease.

"Support" has proved to be very meaningful to me during my cancer journey. Receiving words of encouragement and hope from my "life net": friends, colleagues, neighbors, old classmates from school and neighbors helped to raise my spirits during down times and kept me focused on the fight to overcome the cancer. I have received support from seemingly long-lost friends that I had not seen or heard from in many, many years. Knowing that they had been through the challenges of cancer gave me more determination to overcome cancer and to return to a more normal life when the cancer is behind me. Prostate cancer is probably the most common form of cancer for males, and I have learned that many of my friends from all sections of my life have been down this path. Their comments and offers of support really resonated with me and made the journey more tolerable. They have been with me each step of the way and that has meant a lot to me. More than they will ever know.

"Living a Meaningful Life" has been a key aspect of my life long before I became a cancer patient. It represents my commitment to helping to make life better for the people I have been blessed to come into contact with through community service projects, students, and colleagues I have worked with/taught during my life. Community service projects have shown me that there are others in this world who are much worse off than I am and who do not have the means to change and improve their lot in life. As a cancer patient, I have realized that many friends in the life net have also made the reluctant journey to fight cancer. As they have reached out to me to buoy my spirits, so too have I tried to pay it forward to offer counsel and support as they faced their challenges. From my former students, not only have I received notes of support, but I have also been provided opportunities to further guide them along their career paths and/or pursuits of graduate study. I have found that such opportunities enhance my life and give it greater meaning. In doing so, I have also enriched my own life.

Bonnie Cashin Farmer

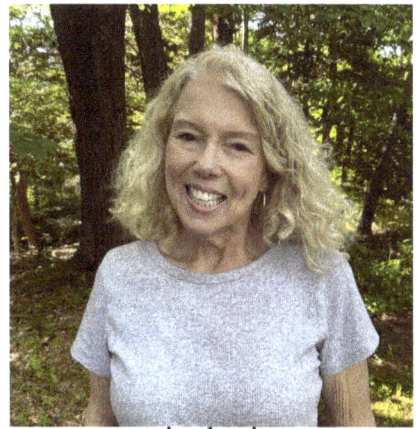

As I reflect upon my lessons learned from this reluctant journey of cancer, I acknowledge that such lessons are many in number and require continual revision of content dependent upon current circumstances. These lessons, well embedded in my chapter writings, all share an interconnectedness within the context of my cancer experience. I leave the reader to choose what lessons might work for them.

One of the lessons of most significance to me is the importance of forming a team of professional healthcare providers to guide the patient or primary caregiver in navigating the complexities of cancer care. A prerequisite for an effective team is the presence of the patient or primary caregiver in the dual role of chief team leader and team member: learning, advocating, problem-solving, evaluating, organizing, and adapting to name a few. As the leader of my team, I remain committed to my ongoing practice of due diligence, patience, and an openness for respect and kindness for self and others. I have been able to develop competent and responsive resources upon which to rely for my care as related to my cancer, decision-making for treatments, and overall well-being.

Underlying all my lessons learned is the acknowledgment that living a meaningful life in the presence of forever choppy waters is a deliberate choice. Such a choice is cultivated by developing one's capacity for the openness to good and inner strength. I am stronger than I ever imagined! During childhood I recall my father would lovingly say that I was a delicate flower on the outside and strong on the inside. As a child I paid little attention and as an adult I often think how right he was so long ago! Recently a friend's spouse received the diagnosis of an advanced stage and potentially deadly cancer. With the fear in her eyes of which I know too well, she said how she wished she could be "strong" like me! With much emotion, I replied that I have been in "training for almost seven years". My personal growth from traveling this reluctant journey has brought me to the acceptance that I am whole, I am most capable, I am human, and I am imperfect. Doing the best to my abilities every day is enough. I remain eternally grateful.

Burt Harres

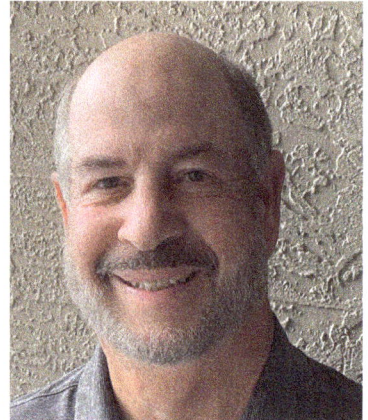

During my life, I have experienced and been cured of various illnesses. When it comes to cancer, there is nothing easy about being diagnosed with it. For most people, cancer is a hard, emotionally, and physically draining reluctant journey through rugged, unfamiliar terrain. Some people, like me, are relatively fortunate because due to early detection, their treatment regimen is not as arduous as someone with a rare or late-stage cancer. I believe that everyone's journey as a cancer patient will be different because there are many forms of cancer as well as diverse methods of treatment. I learned the following three lessons on my journey as a cancer patient:

1. Early detection, screening, and diagnosis have been proven to significantly improve patient survival rates and quality of life, as well as to significantly reduce the cost and complexity of cancer treatment. The majority of cancers are amenable to early detection. When a cancer is detected at an early stage—and when coupled with appropriate treatment—the chance of survival beyond 5 years is higher than when detected at a later stage.

2. For many cancer patients and their families, the experience of cancer is intensely stressful. Accepting support is important for most cancer patients during their illness and can be gained from different people and services. The American Cancer Society (1-800-227-2345 cancer.org) is available 24 hours a day, seven days a week, to help guide a cancer patient with various treatment and support options.

3. Hope is not wishful thinking. Holding on to hope and wishful thinking, a form of denial, are not the same. Denial means that one is avoiding reality and refusing to admit the truth. Having hope may help ease overwhelming doubts and fears. Hope is realistic. Hope is being honest with oneself. Hope requires some form of action so that cancer patients can be honest with their current situations while still looking forward to favorable, future outcomes.

Cherie LaFlamme Genua

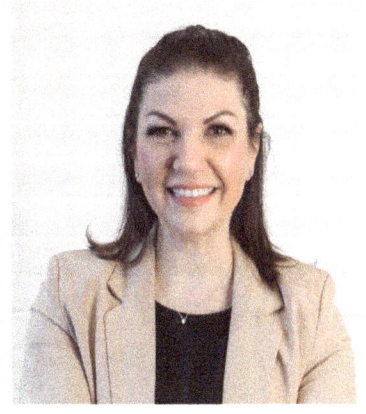

For me, I found the topics of "Being a Cancer Patient," "Hope," and "Living a Meaningful Life" to be cathartic as I looked back upon my breast cancer diagnosis, treatment, and post-cancer journey. Although I am in remission, cancer rears its head often. It tries to remind me of a dark, terrifying, and lonely time in my life but, oftentimes, it falls short. And although being a cancer patient was scary (due to the unknown) and isolating (because it seemed like my life was put on pause while the rest of the world kept spinning), it served to teach me that people—close family and friends, acquaintances, coworkers, and even my social media network—are a cornerstone of support and moving forward. My support system reminded me that someone out there was thinking about me and praying for me to make it through another day, another week, and another month. And as crazy as it seems, I felt that support and it guided me towards healing.

I am so much more than my cancer diagnosis, which is apparent as I try my best to live a meaningful life. By focusing on the things I have—a wonderful husband, supportive family, and friends, fulfilling work, and a spirit that can't be broken—I am able to see the silver lining in all of the hardships I had to endure from getting diagnosed with cancer at the age of 34. I have learned how to go easier on myself as I navigate my post-cancer journey. Yes, I stumble and make mistakes. Sure, I cry out of frustration when I'm getting an MRI and others are enjoying a day at the beach. And, yeah, I sometimes ignore the voice in the back of my head that tells me the back pain I'm experiencing is most likely from exercising or aging, perhaps, and not from a recurrence. Thoughts like this sometimes take over, making me anxious, afraid, and angry, but I try to push them aside and continue living. After all, I am just a human being trying to forge ahead and apply the lessons learned during my cancer journey to the rest of my life. A life that is meaningful and filled with happiness, love, patience, and experiences… not things.

Speaking of living, cancer taught me many things about life, mostly that it is precious. Tell your loved ones how much they mean to you, laugh with them about the memories, or go on that trip you've been wanting to take. Tomorrow is never promised—no matter if we are living with a cancer diagnosis or not. It's up to us to live our lives in such a way that we are not regretful of our past, and instead, hopeful for our futures.

Welcome to the Curry family. Got an idea for a book? Contact Curry Brothers Marketing and Publishing Group, LLC. We are not satisfied until your publishing dreams come true. We specialize in all genres of books, especially religion, leadership, family history, poetry, and children's literature. There is an African Proverb that confirms, *"When an elder dies, a library closes."* We advise, be careful who tells your family history. Are their values your family's values? Our staff will navigate you through the entire publishing process, and we take pride in going the extra mile by exceeding your publishing goals.

Improving the world one book at a time!

Curry Brothers Publishing, LLC
PO Box 247
Haymarket, VA 20168
(719) 466-7518 & (615) 347-9124
Visit us at *www.currybrotherspublishing.com*

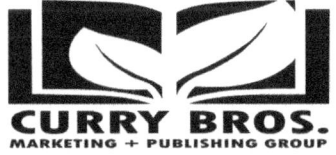

www.ingramcontent.com/pod-product-compliance
Lightning Source LLC
Chambersburg PA
CBHW040420100526
44589CB00021B/2766